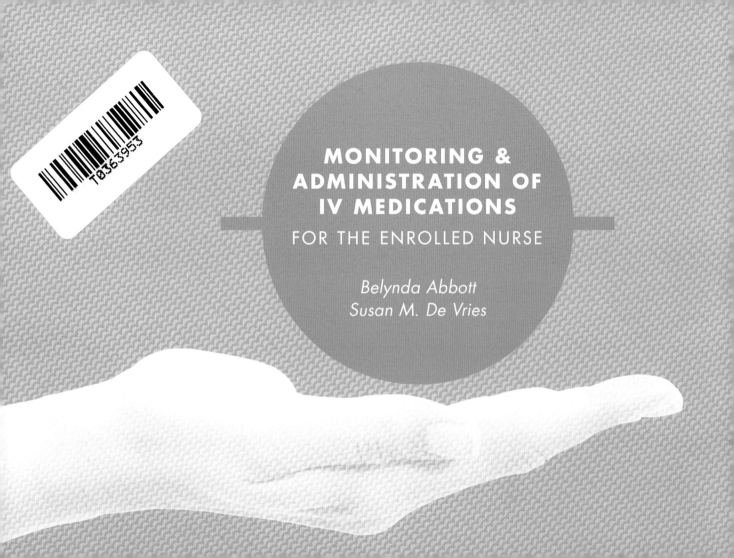

MONITORING & ADMINISTRATION OF IV MEDICATIONS

FOR THE ENROLLED NURSE

Belynda Abbott
Susan M. De Vries

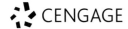
CENGAGE

Monitoring and Administration of IV Medications for the Enrolled Nurse
1st Edition
Belynda Abbott
Susan M. De Vries

Publishing manager: Dorothy Chiu
Senior publishing editor: Sophie Kaliniecki
Developmental editor: Tharaha Richards
Project editors: Michaela Skelly & Amelia Fellows
Art direction: Danielle Maccarone
Cover designer: Emilie Pfitzner (Everyday Ambitions)
Text designer: Norma Van Rees
Editor: Jill Pope
Proofreader: Julie Wicks
Indexer: Julie King
Permissions/Photo researcher: Q2A Media
Cover: iStockphoto/AntonioGuillem
Typeset by MPS Limited

Any URLs contained in this publication were checked for currency during the production process. Note, however, that the publisher cannot vouch for the ongoing currency of URLs.

This first edition published in 2016

NOTE TO THE READER
The publisher does not make any representations, warranties or guarantees regarding any of the products, procedures or treatments described in this publication and does not perform any independent analysis in connection with any of the product information contained in this publication. The publisher expressly disclaims any obligation to obtain and include information other than the information provided to it by the manufacturer of those products and does not make any representations, warranties or guarantees of any kind, including but not limited to, any warranty that the products, instructions or activities described in this publication are of merchantable quality.
The reader is warned to consider and adopt all safety precautions that might be indicated by the activities described in this publication and to avoid all potential hazards. Particularly to note is that the clinical cases used are examples for the purpose of teaching IV administrations and that clinical use of certain medicines and therapeutic regimens may change or not be suitable in all cases. This book is an IV administrations text and is not to be substituted for a pharmacology or medicine administration guide. Readers are not to use the clinical cases or treatment plans for actual patient care beyond their scope as aids in determining IV procedures and protocols. By following the instructions contained in this publication, the reader willingly assumes all risks associated with such activities and instructions. The publisher shall not be liable for any special, consequential, or exemplary damages resulting, in whole or part, from the readers' use of, or reliance upon, the material described in this publication.

For product information and technology assistance,
        in Australia call 1300 790 853;
        in New Zealand call 0800 449 725

For permission to use material from this text or product, please email
aust.permissions@cengage.com

National Library of Australia Cataloguing-in-Publication Data
Creator: Abbott, Belynda, author.
Title: Monitoring and Administration of IV Medications for the Enrolled Nurse
        Belynda Abbott and Susan M. De Vries.
ISBN: 9780170261517 (paperback)
Subjects: Nursing--Study and teaching.
        Drugs--Administration--Study and teaching.
        Injections, Intravenous--Australia.
        nursing assessment
Other Creators/Contributors: De Vries, Susan, M., author.
Dewey Number: 610.73071094

Cengage Learning Australia
Level 7, 80 Dorcas Street
South Melbourne, Victoria Australia 3205

For learning solutions, visit cengage.com.au

Printed in China by 1010 Printing International Limited.
3 4 5 6 7 8 26 25 24

BRIEF CONTENTS

CONTENTS

ABOUT THE BOOK

Administering and monitoring IV medications in the nursing environment is part of the curriculum of the national Enrolled-Division 2 nursing program as determined within the Australian Qualifications Framework (AQF). The knowledge and skills that are obtained in the unit of competence require practice and application in the clinical setting. The book aims to clarify and apply information to assist those working in this area of enrolled nursing practice. This book will be your supportive companion for your student and professional practice.

Health professionals are taught medication theory and calculations but may require step-by-step instructions related to exactly *how* a medication is administered. *Monitoring and Administration of IV Medications for the Enrolled Nurse* provides these instructions and realistic clinical application scenarios.

This text is positioned within the truths of clinical practice by using real-life cases, examples and medicines. National guidelines and initiatives such as those found within the Australian Commission on Safety and Quality in Health Care are referenced and used for guidance in this high-risk area of medication administration. This assists students and practitioners to increase their familiarity with the best practices relating to administering IV medications and to be able to source the latest details.

It is beyond the scope of this text to act as a pharmacology resource or medicine administration guide; other relevant texts are needed for these purposes. This book only offers a supportive guide relating to the realities of administering IV medications for enrolled nurses and encourages the reader to access local policies and procedures, other texts and local legislative requirements.

Monitoring and Administration of IV Medications for the Enrolled Nurse introduces a national view of the scheduling of medications. It provides clarity relating to the various laws and regulations around this aspect of enrolled nursing practice. There is continuous reference to potential emergency situations with relevant related images. The various infusion devices are discussed and contextualised.

There are distinctive approaches to assisting with the placement of an IV line. This text includes step-by-step instructions and images starting from 'priming the line' and extending to mixing the most common IV medications and giving them safely. The text also incorporates special-area scenarios and guidance, which include the older adult and the child. Questions at the end of each chapter encourage the reader to engage in clinical thinking tasks related to this important area of clinical practice.

This text may be read from 'front to back', or the reader may choose to skip to the section relevant to them and use the examples to guide learning and practice. It would be advisable for readers to read through the general chapters first before the specialist areas but this is not strictly required. Each chapter explains the main concepts and gives clinical examples. There are tip boxes throughout to guide the reader with clinical know-how. It is hoped that you will enjoy reading and using *Monitoring and Administration of IV Medications for the Enrolled Nurse* in your learning and clinical practice.

ABOUT THE AUTHORS

Belynda J. Abbott, RN, BN, GDipClinEd, Cert IV TAE, FACN, is a Nurse Educator at the Princess Alexandra Hospital in Brisbane. Belynda has worked as a Clinical Nurse and Nurse Educator at both the Royal Brisbane and Women's Hospital and the Royal Darwin Hospital for many years. She has experience in neurosciences, orthopaedics, infectious diseases, hyperbaric nursing, surgical and general medicine. Belynda is the key contact for the Brisbane region of the Australian College of Nursing and has a passion for mentoring and guiding the next generation of nurses. She is committed to providing leadership within the nursing profession and is passionate about education and building capacity to provide optimal patient care. Belynda has extensive knowledge and expertise in clinical and organisational planning, implementation and evaluation of education, training and development initiatives.

Susan M. De Vries, RN, DipAppSci(NEd), BA, MPH, Cert IV TAE, FACN, is currently a sessional lecturer at the Australian Catholic University's Banyo Campus in Brisbane. Sue also has managed and delivered teaching in the Diploma of Nursing, providing educational leadership and preparation for enrolled nurses. She currently works as a sessional registered nurse in general practice and has had past experience in intensive care, orthopaedics, post-anaesthetic care, day surgery and endoscopy. She has been an education manager in residential and community aged care. She has experience teaching in an RN program at Central Queensland University in Rockhampton and Griffith University in Brisbane. Sue has also worked as a nurse researcher across various projects. Sue has a strong interest in teaching and learning, evidence-based practice, and guiding and mentoring the next generation of nurses.

ACKNOWLEDGEMENTS

This book would not have been possible without the support of our family and colleagues. Thank you to our external reviewers for your valuable feedback and advice on each of the chapters. Also a big thank you to the Cengage team, especially Tharaha Richards (development editor) and Sophie Kaliniecki (publishing editor) for their patience, expertise and knowledge in supporting the development of our first textbook.

From Belynda: I would like to thank my husband Steven and my two beautiful children, Sophy and Luke, for their support and encouragement. I would also like to thank my parents and my family for helping in the many ways that they do. I could not have done this without the support, guidance and friendship of my mentors Dr Catriona Booker and Susan M. De Vries, RN: these two amazing nurse leaders have guided and moulded me into the nurse I am today. I would also like to say a big thank you to Bradley Wessling, RN, who introduced me to the concept of writing this textbook. To all of my nursing colleagues, both RN and EN, this book is for you to assist with providing optimal and safe patient care.

From Susan: Firstly, a special thanks to my husband John for his patience and thoughtfulness. I would also like to acknowledge my nursing colleagues who have freely provided their experience and expertise from their various workplaces. Reflections and comments about the essential day-to-day work they do have informed this work and made it richer. Many thanks also go to my friends Lesley Scheelings and Eva Coggins who have given thoughtful input within their areas of expertise. Finally, I would like to acknowledge all of my students, past and present: some now practising as ENs or RNs or NPs. Your work is the glue that holds our healthcare system together.

Belynda Abbott and Susan M. De Vries

Cengage Learning would like to thank the following lecturers who provided feedback on the plans for this text in the early stages of its development or reviewed draft chapters, as well as those who provided anonymous feedback:

Tracey Christian – The Gordon Institute of TAFE
Mike Shearsmith – Challenger Institute of Technology
Narelle Howelle – Tasmania Polytechnic
Anne Moates – Chisholm Institute
Gregory Furness – University of Ballarat
Jennifer Hill – Kyabram Community Learning Centre
Jennifer Lohan – Australian College of Nursing
Kristine Sonter – Wodonga TAFE
Marie Chittleborough – EQUALS International
Kaye McDonald – Tasmanian Polytechnic
Suzanne McArthur – Advance TAFE
Lindsay Bava – Kangan Institute
Meryl Chaffey – TAFE NSW New England Institute
Gayle Watson – Central Institute of Technology

Guide to the text

As you read this text you will find a number of features in every chapter to enhance your study of the monitoring and administration of IV medications.

FEATURES WITHIN CHAPTERS

EXAMPLE

Example boxes illustrate key concepts throughout the text.

> **EXAMPLE**
>
> **Schedule 2 poisons**
>
> Schedule 2 poisons include mild analgesics, anti-inflammatory agents, topical antifungals, cough and cold preparations, some antihistamines.
>
> Department of Health Therapeutic Goods Administration (2011); Koutoukidis, Stainton and Hughson (2013)

CASE STUDY

Case studies showcase real-life scenarios, to make your learning more meaningful.

> **CASE STUDY**
>
> **IV medications for treating sepsis**
>
> Mrs Andrews is an 86-year-old lady who has been admitted to the hospital from an aged care facility with sepsis secondary to a urinary tract infection and dehydration. Mrs Andrews is prescribed 1 litre of 0.9% normal saline IV at 125 mL/h. The doctor has also prescribed ciprofloxacin 400 mg 8 hourly.
>
> 1 What is the safest way of administering the IV fluids? What IV equipment will you be required to use?

TIP BOX

Tip boxes emphasise the key clinical concepts you will need to consider.

TIP BOX

Understanding scope of practice
A nurse's scope of practice covers:
- the context in which they practise
- the patients' health needs
- their level of education (completing approved educational requirements)
- their qualification and competency to administer IV medicines.

 Legal/ethics icons appear throughout the text to help you identify essential ethical prerequisites and legal requirements.

 Easily cross reference with *Essential Clinical Skills* 3rd edn, using the **Essential Clinical Skills icon**.

ACTIVITY

Test your understanding of important concepts and practise calculations with the **activities** throughout each chapter.

ACTIVITY

Using abbreviations
Search for and find the document above by the Australian Commission on Safety and Quality in Health Care (Arcus et al. 2011). Go to 'Table 2: Acceptable Terms and Abbreviations'. Then do the following:
1 Copy the commonly used abbreviations and their related meaning from Table 3.1 in this chapter.

 Easily cross reference with *Foundations of Nursing: Enrolled/Division 2 Nurses* using the **Foundations of Nursing icon**.

END OF CHAPTER FEATURES

At the end of the chapter you will find:
- a summary of key points
- review questions.

END OF BOOK FEATURES

At the end of the book you will find:
- appendices covering medication-related legislative requirements for New Zealand and Australia, and a summary of intravenous care
- additional review questions and answers
- a glossary of key terms from throughout the text.

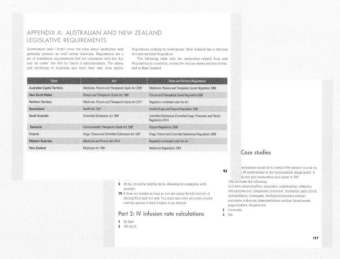

SUMMARY

Within this chapter the following concepts and issues related to IV medication have been covered:
- A bolus is a common form of administration method whereby a small volume of IV medication or fluid is carefully pushed directly into the PIVC via the IV access port.
- IV lines that are compatible with electronic infusion pumps are considered a safer option than gravity-fed lines because they decrease the risk of both air embolus and also the infusion being administered too quickly.
- Burettes can be used between the bag or bottle of IV medication or fluid and the IV line.
- The three types of pumps commonly used within the healthcare environment are volumetric pumps, syringe pumps and the PCAs.

- If a patient requires two or more IV medications to be administered, an IV piggyback/tandem approach can be used.
- It is a part of an EN's scope of practice to monitor, care and maintain the safe and effective use of PIVCs and infusion equipment.
- An EN needs to recognise signs and symptoms of a compromised PIVC and visually check the insertion site and palpate the surrounding skin at least every 8 hours, before and after every intermittent infusion and hourly for continuous infusions.
- It is essential that the principles of ANTT and the World Health Organization guidelines around hand hygiene are clearly understood and adopted.

REVIEW QUESTIONS

1. What is the difference between infiltration and extravasation?
2. Name the four different types of phlebitis.
3. What is the nursing management of inflammation and infection of a PIVC site?
4. What are the three most commonly used infusion pumps?
5. What principles should be adopted to prevent healthcare associated infections of the PIVC?

APPENDIX A: AUSTRALIAN AND NEW ZEALAND LEGISLATIVE REQUIREMENTS

Government laws ('Acts') cover the rules about medicines (and generally patients as well) across Australia. Regulations are a set of mandatory requirements that are consistent with the Act and 'sit under' the Act for clarity of administration. The states and territories of Australia also have their own Acts and/or

Regulations relating to medicines too. New Zealand has a national Act and national Regulation.

The following table lists the medication-related Acts and Regulations in Australia, across the various states and territories, and in New Zealand.

State	Act	State and Territory Regulations
Australian Capital Territory	Medicines, Poisons and Therapeutic Goods Act 2008	Medicines, Poisons and Therapeutic Goods Regulation 2008
New South Wales	Poisons and Therapeutic Goods Act 1966	Poisons and Therapeutic Goods Regulation 2008
Northern Territory	Medicines, Poisons and Therapeutic Goods Act 2012	Regulation contained under the Act
Queensland	Health Act 1937	Health (Drugs and Poisons) Regulation 1996
South Australia	Controlled Substances Act 1984	Controlled Substances (Controlled Drugs, Precursors and Plants) Regulations 2014
Tasmania	Commonwealth, Therapeutic Goods Act 1989	Poisons Regulations 2008
Victoria	Drugs, Poisons and Controlled Substances Act 1981	Drugs, Poisons and Controlled Substances Regulations 2006
Western Australia	Medicines and Poisons Act 2014	Regulation contained under the Act
New Zealand	Medicines Act 1981	Medicines Regulations 1984

95

Case studies

...medicine would be to check if the patient is now on ...n IV medication in the incompatible drugs listed. If ...do not give medication and report to RN.

This includes the following:
Aciclovir, aminophylline, ampicillin, azathioprine, cefepime, chloramphenicol, citanazepam, furosemid, fluconazole, ganciclovir, indomethacin, lansoprem, methylprednisolone sodium succinate, nafcisone, phenobarbitone, sodium bicarbonate, voriconazole, disoproxine

2. 3 minutes
3. Yes

9. 40 mL (could be slightly more, allowing for expansion with powder)
10. It does not matter as long as you are using the full amount of diluting fluid and not less. You must also have accurate control over the period of time it takes to be infused.

Part 2: IV infusion rate calculations

1. 34 dpm
2. 300 mL/h

117

Guide to the online resources

FOR THE INSTRUCTOR

Cengage Learning is pleased to provide you with resources that will help you prepare your lectures and assessments. These teaching tools are accessible via http://login.cengage.com.

INSTRUCTOR'S MANUAL
The instructor's manual includes:
- solutions to problems and cases
- additional scenarios.

TEST BANK
A test bank of questions, covering each of the units of competency as well as the learning objectives and key topics, has been prepared for your use. The questions are available in Word file format and can be uploaded directly into your Learning Management System or customised to meet your students' learning requirements.

POWERPOINT™ PRESENTATIONS
Use the chapter-by-chapter PowerPoint presentations to enhance your lecture presentations and to reinforce the key principles of your subject, or for student handouts.

ARTWORK FROM THE TEXT
Add the digital files of graphs, pictures and flowcharts into your course management system, use them within student handouts or copy them into lecture presentations.

MAPPING GRID
A detailed competency mapping grid shows you how the core competencies for *Administer and monitor intravenous medication in the nursing environment* are covered in this book.

FOR THE STUDENT

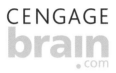

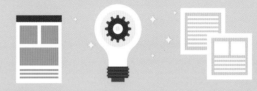

Visit the Monitoring and Administration of IV Medications for the Enrolled Nurse companion website. You'll find:

- quizzes
- competency mapping
- flashcards
- crosswords.

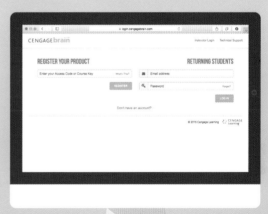

1 ROLE OF THE HEALTHCARE TEAM IN THE ADMINISTRATION OF IV MEDICATIONS

LEARNING OBJECTIVES

After completing this chapter, you will be able to:

- outline the legal requirements and practice parameters of the EN/Div 2 nurse in relation to IV medications
- recognise the various schedules within medication regulation
- understand the various types of intravenous (IV) administration in relation to scope of practice and legal requirements
- identify, alert and implement medical emergency management within the context of IV medication administration
- describe and understand the anatomy and physiology in relation to IV medication administration.

Introduction

Intravenous (IV) medication administration within the enrolled nurse's scope of practice has many complexities, ranging from legislation and standards of practice to local policies and procedures that are the foundations to ensuring patient/client safety.

It is important to explore and understand these complexities as an integral member of the healthcare team.

Legal requirements

The **enrolled nurse** (EN) is accountable and responsible for their own **scope of practice** and must ensure that they adhere to principles of delegation and supervision set out in the professional practice framework approved by the Nursing and Midwifery Board of Australia (NMBA), a national board of the Australian Health Practitioners Registration Authority (AHPRA), to protect themselves and their patients/clients. There are components that influence the EN's scope of practice that will allow them to administer IV medication.

TIP BOX

Understanding scope of practice

A nurse's scope of practice covers:

- the context in which they practise
- the patients' health needs
- their level of education (completing approved educational requirements)
- their qualification and competency to administer IV medicines.

- their compliance with local policies, procedures and protocols in order to work within an employer's processes and guidelines.

  Nursing and Midwifery Board of Australia (2007)

 Legal requirements are broad, whereas local policies and procedures are often specific to a work environment.

Registration

Since 2010, the national nursing register (a public register) places a notation next to the individual EN's name stating 'Does not hold Board-approved qualification in administration of medicines' if the relevant units of study have not been completed and the EN is therefore not qualified to administer medicines. (Nursing and Midwifery Board of Australia 2014) It is the EN's responsibility to ensure that they practise within their scope of practice in order to protect the public and themselves. It is ultimately the EN's responsibility to inform the NMBA if they have not completed relevant units of study and therefore require a notation on their licence. (Australian Nursing and Midwifery Council 2002)

TIP BOX

Essential units of study

Current essential units of study for administration of IV medications in the Health Training Package include the following:
- Analyse health information
- Administer and monitor medications in the work environment
- Contribute to work health and safety processes
- Comply with infection control policies and procedures
- Contribute to the complex nursing care of patients.

Elective units of study for administration of medicines in the Health Training Package currently include the following:
- Administer and monitor intravenous medication in the nursing environment.

Nursing and Midwifery Board of Australia (2014)

TABLE 1.1 Enrolled Nurses' Medication Endorsement with AHPRA: Before and after 2010

Prior to 2010	Since 2010
There were both ENs (Enrolled Nurses) and EENs (Endorsed Enrolled Nurses) practising.	Now there are only ENs practising.
There was a medication unit in the Enrolled Nursing course of study that was an elective. This meant only some ENs had this unit and then had the special title of EEN.	Now all courses of study for Enrolled Nursing include a medication unit (but not an IV medication unit). This is under review.
The regulators (AHPRA and NMBA) identified on the register of ENs which ENs were medication endorsed – and this showed with the registration.	Now the regulators only make a notation if the Enrolled Nurse does NOT have medication units. This is usually for ENs who have completed their course in the pre-2010 era and have not later completed the unit of competence.

The tip box shows that currently the administration and monitoring of IV medication is an elective unit. Therefore, if an EN has a notation that states that they do not hold Board-approved qualification in administration of medicines they can not administer IV medications. An EN can expand their scope of practice and administer IV medication once they have completed the appropriate elective unit of study and their aligning prerequisite components in accordance with the Health Training Package and are deemed competent in the area. (Nursing and Midwifery Board of Australia 2014)

 For more-detailed nursing legal and ethical information, see Chapter 4 in *Foundations of Nursing*.

Scheduling of medications

Prescription medication, agricultural poisons and research drugs are governed by local state and territory drugs and poisons legislation. The EN without a notation who is deemed competent to administer medications must adhere to their scope of practice and these governing laws and regulations from a national and local level. These laws and regulations include scheduling, which is a national classification system that controls how medicines and poisons are applied for sale, supply, storage, dispensing and labelling. (Department of Health Therapeutic Goods Administration 2011; Koutoukidis, Stainton & Hughson 2013) Public health and safety is very important when medicines and poisons are classified, therefore the schedule is in accordance with the level of regulatory control over the availability of the medicine or poison to the public.

As there is no national medicines and poisons schedule for Australia, the Poisons Standard has the overarching decision making regarding the classification for inclusion in the relevant legislation of state and territory law. (Department of Health Therapeutic Goods Administration 2011; Koutoukidis Stainton & Hughson 2013)

There are five schedules that are important for ENs to know and understand when administering and/or checking medications.

Schedule 2 poisons

Medicines in this schedule are labelled 'Pharmacy medicine'. These medicines are available to the public for ailments or conditions that do not require medical attention and can be obtained only from a pharmacy. If a pharmacy service is unavailable, a person must be licenced to sell Schedule 2 poisons.

EXAMPLE

Schedule 2 poisons
Schedule 2 poisons include mild analgesics, anti-inflammatory agents, topical antifungals, cough and cold preparations, some antihistamines.
Department of Health Therapeutic Goods Administration (2011); Koutoukidis, Stainton and Hughson (2013)

Schedule 3 poisons

Schedule 3 medicines are labelled as 'Pharmacy only medicine' and are only available to the public from a pharmacist, or a medical, dental or veterinary practitioner, without the need for a prescription. Professional advice is required for the safe use of these medicines. Storage must not be accessible to the public. The pharmacist may require identification to dispense these medicines.

> **EXAMPLE**
>
> **Schedule 3 poisons**
> Schedule 3 poisons include codeine, topical corticosteroids and metered dose bronchodilators.
>
> Department of Health Therapeutic Goods Administration (2011);
> Koutoukidis, Stainton and Hughson (2013)

Schedule 4 poisons

Medicines in this schedule are labelled 'Prescription only medicine' and are only used or supplied under a prescription from a medical, dental or veterinary practitioner. Storage is within a dispensary. Nurse practitioners, optometrists and podiatrists with the appropriate qualifications may prescribe a limited range of Schedule 4 medicines.

> **EXAMPLE**
>
> **Schedule 4 poisons**
> Schedule 4 poisons include antibiotics, insulin, antidepressants, cardiovascular drugs and vaccines.
>
> Department of Health Therapeutic Goods Administration (2011);
> Koutoukidis, Stainton and Hughson (2013)

Restricted Schedule 4 poisons

Restricted Schedule 4 poisons are liable to abuse and may cause dependence. Medicines must be stored in a locked cabinet with records kept for two years.

> **EXAMPLE**
>
> **Restricted Schedule 4 poisons**
> Restricted Schedule 4 poisons include benzodiazepines, hypnotic sedatives and opioid-like analgesics.
>
> Department of Health Therapeutic Goods Administration (2011);
> Koutoukidis, Stainton and Hughson (2013)

Schedule 8 poisons

Schedule 8 poisons are labelled as a 'Controlled drug'. They are medicines or substances that may produce addiction or dependence. Prescriptions are only valid for three months. Medicines must be stored in a locked cabinet, with records kept for three years. It is illegal to possess these drugs without authority.

> **EXAMPLE**
>
> **Schedule 8 poisons**
> Schedule 8 poisons include opioids, and central nervous system (CNS) stimulants.
>
> Department of Health Therapeutic Goods Administration (2011);
> Koutoukidis, Stainton and Hughson (2013)

You must know which schedule various drugs belong to.

ACTIVITY

Generic names of medicines

List five medicines from each schedule. Use generic names.

Legal requirements of IV administration

When administering IV medication, it is important for the EN to understand:

- the various types of IV administration
- their own scope of practice
- the legal requirements in accordance with the NMBA and the employer's local policies and guidelines.

Understanding local **policies, procedures** and **guidelines** is essential, as each health facility governs EN scope of practice and the administration of IV medications differently. It is important for the EN to familiarise themselves with their local policies, procedures and guidelines by accessing these resources via the health facility. As the EN you are accountable for your own scope of practice and therefore it is important to seek the information from a legal/endorsed written source rather than asking a colleague. This is to protect your patients/clients and your registration from potential unsafe practices.

Due to the complexity of the information and regulation surrounding medications, you need well-developed **information literacy** skills. According to the Information Literacy Competency Standards for Higher Education of the American Library Association (2009), a person has information literacy when they are able to:

- make a decision about the type of information needed
- obtain access to required information in a timely and efficient manner
- critically evaluate the information to determine its source and suitability
- use suitable information effectively in their personal knowledge base to achieve goals
- act upon an understanding of the social, economic, legal and ethical considerations around the use of information.

Because there is a large amount of information available today, you must be able to understand how to determine the quality of information accessed when searching the Internet. Medications have both chemical and commercial names and this can be confusing. This is a safety risk.

 It is important to use information from a formal, written source relating to legal issues. Word of mouth from a friend or colleague can be misinterpreted, out of date or incorrect.

TIP BOX

Information literacy

Some key questions to consider when searching for information related to IV medications include the following:

- Is the information from a reputable website such as a government department, a university department or a well-regarded association in the community?
- Is the information from Australia (or the country where you are practising)? If it is not from Australia, does it apply to the Australian healthcare system and culture? Adding the search term 'Australia' to your search will narrow down results to Australian regulations and frameworks.
- Is there a financial incentive for sales of medication within the website? Is its sole purpose one of promotion of a product rather than unbiased information?

CASE STUDY

Scope of practice

Frank, a 68-year-old man, was admitted to the emergency department with an infected diabetic foot wound. He has a history of diabetes, hypertension and osteoarthritis. Frank was transferred to a medical ward for IV antibiotics, wound management and close observation. As the EN caring for Frank on the evening shift you notice on the National Inpatient Medication Chart that he has IV Timentin (ticarcillin plus clavulanic acid) 3.1 g 6 hourly prescribed.

1   As the EN can you give this IV medication?
2   Is it within your scope of practice? Why?
3   What is essential for the EN to know and understand prior to any IV administration?

Table 1.2 gives a brief explanation of the different types of IV lines that you might use in the healthcare environment.

TABLE 1.2 Understanding IV access

IV method	Explanation
Peripherally inserted vascular catheters (PIVCs)	Peripheral IVs are the most commonly used. They are a short-term vascular access device. They are small, flexible catheters that are inserted into a peripheral vein.
Central venous access devices (CVADs) • non-tunnelled • tunnelled • peripherally inserted central catheter (PICC) • implanted ports	CVADs are commonly used for short- or long-term therapy. They are placed in the chest, neck, arm or groin with the catheter inserted into the veins of the central venous system, such as the superior vena cava or inferior vena cava.

Nosek and Trendel-Leader (2013)

To understand the legal requirements regarding IV regulation you must understand the NMBA Nursing practice decisions summary guide. Identify the patient's needs, reflect on your scope of practice and your nursing practice standards, consider the context in which you practise and your organisational support and policies. After these considerations you will be able to decide if you have the required knowledge, skill, authority and ability to administer IV medications.

You must understand the difference between law and organisational policy. As you will have covered in the unit 'Apply legal and ethical parameters to nursing practice', each level of government has laws and responsibilities. It is useful to review this with regard to your administration of IV medications. **Figure 1.1** illustrates the relationship between the various laws, regulations and local organisational policies, procedures and guidelines.

FIGURE 1.1 The relationship between laws, regulations and organisational policies

Relevant national, state and local government Acts
Example: *Queensland Health Act, 1937*

↓

Regulations arise out of the various Acts
Example: Queensland Health (Drugs and Poisons) Regulation, 1996

↓

Organisations interpret these acts and develop organisational policies
Example: Ramsey Health Care, in some areas, has its own 'in-house' courses for ENs and various medications in conjunction with a relevant training organisation and local policies. See announcement in the newsletter at http://www.ramsayhealth.com/news/documents/TRW_08_Dec.pdf

An EN needs to be familiar with the different forms of access discussed and to understand how to care and monitor each of these forms. Each health facility has different governing policies, procedures and guidelines around scope of practice and the EN's scope regarding these forms of access.

The EN's role in a medical emergency

The role of the EN within a medical emergency with IV medication administration is to identify, alert and implement emergency actions for acute and delayed adverse drug reactions. One type of adverse drug reaction that can have severe consequences for the patient is anaphylaxis, which is a rapid-onset allergic reaction that can potentially cause death if not acted on quickly. Chapter 2 contains more detail of the factors that influence IV medication actions.

First and foremost it is essential to risk manage and prevent adverse reactions. Chapter 2 deals in more depth with anaphylactic and adverse reactions, and Chapter 3 describes safely preparing, administering and recording IV medications.

In an emergency event where a patient is identified as having an anaphylactic reaction, stop the causative agent immediately. It is important to keep the IV in situ and call for help or assistance. Ensure that you are following your facilities policies and guidelines with emergency management. Maintain airway support by providing a head tilt. See **Figure 1.2**. You may require setting up for further IV access and setting up for the administration of IM or IV adrenaline. Place the patient in the supine or recovery position and elevate legs as tolerated. (Brown, Mullins & Gold 2006)

FIGURE 1.2 Chin lift and head tilt

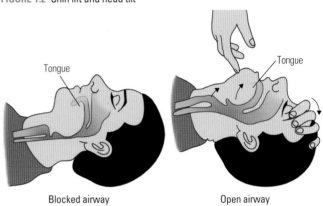

Tongue

Tongue

Blocked airway   Open airway

Introduction of anatomy and physiology

Intravenous can be defined as 'situated within, performed within, occurring within, or administered by entering a vein'. (http://www.merriam-webster.com/medical/intravenous) The fastest way of delivering fluids and medications throughout the body is by the IV route. (Nosek & Trendel-Leader 2013) Intravenous access is required for various reasons including:

- administration of medications
- administration of fluids
- administration of blood products

- emergency administration of medications
- administration of diagnostic substances (e.g. contrast).

To administer into a **vein**, an access device such as a peripheral intravenous catheter (PIVC) or central venous access device (CVAD) can be inserted by a trained and competent health professional. The type of device is determined by the required treatment as discussed in Table 1.2 on page 7. For example, if the patient requires short-term IV antibiotics, a PIVC would be suitable whereas for a patient on long-term chemotherapy a CVAD would be suitable.

The difference between veins and arteries is that veins converge into larger vessels and carry blood toward the heart, whereas arteries branch into smaller arteries (also known as arterioles) and carry blood away from the heart. Veins (except for pulmonary veins) contain dark red blood, have a slow blood return, are superficial, contain valves and multiple veins drain an area. Arteries (except for pulmonary arteries) contain bright red blood, have a rapid blood return, are deeply located, have no valves and a single artery supplies an area. The main veins that are used for IV medication administration are the superficial veins in the hand and forearm. (Alexander et al. 2010) Refer to **Table 1.3** and **Figure 1.3** for the anatomical position of veins located in the hand and the forearm.

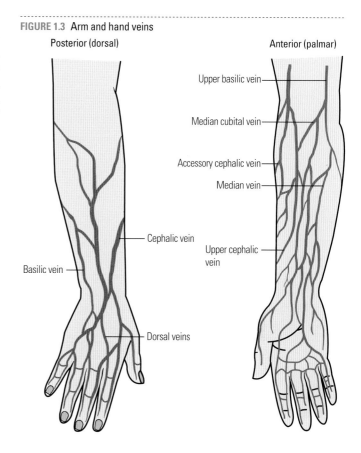

FIGURE 1.3 Arm and hand veins

Posterior (dorsal)

Anterior (palmar)

Upper basilic vein

Median cubital vein

Accessory cephalic vein

Median vein

Upper cephalic vein

Cephalic vein

Basilic vein

Dorsal veins

TABLE 1.3 Veins of the hand and arm

Veins of the hand and forearm	Position
Dorsal metacarpal veins	Most distal veins. Located on top of the hand
Cephalic vein	Lateral (thumb) side of the arm
Basilic vein	Along the medial (little finger) side of the arm
Median cubital vein	In the antecubital fossa
Median vein	Along the underside of the arm and joins the basilic or median cubital vein
Accessory cephalic vein	Branches off the cephalic vein on the top of the forearm
Upper cephalic vein	On the upper arm, lateral side
Upper basilic vein	On the upper arm, medial side

Alexander et al. (2010)

Arteries and veins have similarities and differences. **Table 1.4** defines the three layers within arteries and veins. Arteries carry blood away from the heart and therefore their vessel walls are strong and elastic. They pulsate and lie deep in the tissue, generally protected by muscle. Veins return de-oxygenated blood to the heart and are generally superficial. Veins do not pulsate. **Figure 1.4** illustrates the structure of the arteries, capillaries and veins.

 For more details about vein location and venepuncture, see page 539 of *Foundations of Nursing* and page 208 of *Essential Clinical Skills* 3rd edn.

TABLE 1.4 The three layers within arteries and veins

Vein layer	Artery layer
Tunica intima/interna • thin layer, which forms valves in veins to prevent backflow	Tunica intima/interna • innermost layer, smooth layer of endothelial cells to maximise blood flow
Tunica media • not as strong or stiff as in arteries, surrounded by an elastic membrane, tendency to distend or collapse as pressure rises and falls	Tunica media • middle layer of muscle, elastic tissue and nerve fibres. Does not collapse
Tunica adventitia/externa • thinner than in arteries	Tunica adventitia/externa • outer layer, supports vessel and is thicker than in veins

FIGURE 1.4 Structure of arteries, capillaries and veins

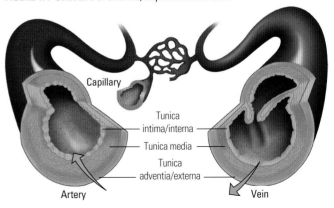

Within this chapter the following concepts and issues related to IV medication have been covered:

- It is a legal requirement of the EN to be accountable and responsible for their own scope of practice and they must adhere to principals of delegation and supervision as set out by the NMBA.
- ENs must understand the governing laws around scheduling of poisons. Schedules 2, 3, 4 and 8 all relate to medicines.
- It is the responsibility of the EN to understand their own scope of practice and the context in which they may practise, which will differ due to different organisational policies.
- The role of the EN within a medical emergency with IV medication administration is to identify, alert and implement emergency actions for acute and delayed adverse drug reactions.
- A sound knowledge and understanding of artery and vein anatomy is essential as an EN.

REVIEW QUESTIONS

1 Name the factors that influence scope of practice for the EN?
2 Name the four schedules that an EN needs to know when administering and/or checking medications.
3 What is the difference between PIVCs and CVADs?
4 As an EN what are the legal guides that are used to determine scope of practice in association with IV access?
5 What are the emergency management steps that are used when dealing with an anaphylactic reaction?
6 Name and locate the various veins of the arm and hand.

LEARNING OBJECTIVES

After completing this chapter, you will be able to:

- apply the principles of pharmacodynamics in nursing practice
- apply the principles of pharmacokinetics in nursing practice
- differentiate between substance incompatibilities and drug interactions and the actions required for both
- relate an understanding of toxicology and its relationship to IV medication administration
- outline the common factors influencing IV medication actions.

Introduction

Across a wide range of healthcare settings, the prescription of IV medications is a decision made by a treating medical practitioner or nurse practitioner, depending on the setting. This treatment has both benefits and risks. These benefits and risks are part of the decision making process for the prescribing practitioner.

The EN also needs to take the benefits and risks into consideration. Various issues, including underpinning scientific knowledge, will inform your practice when monitoring and administering any IV medications.

Pharmacodynamics

Pharmacodynamics has been defined as 'the study ... of the effects of drugs on the body'. (Golan, Tashjian & Armstrong 2012, p. 26) Simply put, pharmacodynamics is what any drug does to the human body.

The majority of drugs act by one of two mechanisms. These are:

- working via various **receptor sites** to promote or inhibit healthy body processes
- interfering with significant processes of the parasites and microbes that can attack the body.

Specific drug actions can be classified into a few main categories:

- stimulating or depressing action in the cells of the body through direct stimulation of a receptor – sometimes described like a key fitting into a lock (e.g. asthma relievers are often 'beta agonists' meaning that they stimulate the beta cells around the lungs telling them to relax; the unintended side effects of jitteriness and tachycardia are from the stimulation of other 'unintended' beta cells in the body)

- blocking action – called **antagonists** when the drug binds the receptor and obstructs it (e.g. some antibiotics work by blocking the synthesis of cell walls of the infecting organism)
- stabilising – acting to keep the environment stable within cells (e.g. propranolol and some other blood pressure medications)
- replacing substances or accumulating them when they need to be held by the body (e.g. insulin acts by replacing the insulin unable to be produced by the body)
- direct destructive chemical reaction that might result in damage or death of cells (e.g. cytotoxics used for cancer)
- beneficial chemical reactions such as free radical scavenging (e.g. vitamin C).

The pharmacologic response of a drug depends on the drug binding to its target (receptor) in the body. The concentration of the drug at the receptor site influences the drug's effect.

Sources: Frandsen and Pennington (2013); National Institute of General Medical Sciences; Merck Sharp & Dohme

ACTIVITY

Learning drug names

IV cephalexin (trade name Keflex) is commonly used as an IV antibiotic when a person has an infection. **Table 2.1** shows the results of an Internet search on 'cephalexin'.

TABLE 2.1 Learning drug names

Generic (chemical) name	Common trade names in Australia	Classification	Group it belongs to	Mode of action
cephalexin	Keflex, Rancef, Ibilex	antibiotic	beta lactam group	inhibits cell wall synthesis of certain infection-causing organisms

Use your information literacy skills (as outlined in Chapter 1) to find the trade names, classification, group and mode of action of the following drugs:

1 metronidazole
2 gentamicin (sometimes spelled gentamycin).

Pharmacokinetics

Pharmacokinetics links with pharmacodynamics. It is 'what the body does to the drug'.

A number of phases occur once a drug enters the body. The acronym LADME will help you learn these phases. It stands for **L**iberation, **A**bsorption, **D**istribution, **M**etabolism and **E**xcretion. The first two phases are pharmacokinetics. The second three phases are pharmacodynamics. See **Table 2.2** which summarises and labels the phases of both pharmacokinetics and pharmacodynamics. For more information on pharmacodynamics and pharmacokinetics, see Merck Manuals.

 For further detailed information about pharmacokinetics, see page 512 of *Foundations of Nursing.*

TABLE 2.2 Phases of pharmacokinetics and pharmacodynamics

	Phase of drug distribution	Description
Pharmacokinetics	Liberation	The releasing of the drug from the form in which it is stored (e.g. in solid oral forms of medications, breaking into smaller particles)
	Absorption	The mechanism by which the medication is taken into the body (e.g. through the skin, the intestine, oral mucosa or, with IV medications, into the blood)
Pharmacodynamics	Distribution	The way the drug behaves as it moves through the body. This action is likely to be faster with IV medications due to direct access into blood stream
	Metabolism	How the medication is converted inside the body, and into what substances
	Excretion	How the medication is eliminated from the body (e.g. via the kidney, skin, breath, gut or a combination)

Merck manual professional edition http://www.merckmanuals.com/professional/clinical_pharmacology/pharmacodynamics/overview_of_pharmacodynamics.html; http://www.merckmanuals.com/professional/clinical_pharmacology/pharmacokinetics/overview_of_pharmacokinetics.html

When you study pharmacokinetics and pharmacodynamics you can follow the course of the drug throughout the body.

With IV medications, the first two phases – liberation and absorption – do not occur as the drug enters the blood stream directly via an IV cannula. This is one of the reasons why IV medications are used frequently in acute situations where the person needs to get medication into their system very quickly.

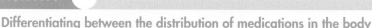

ACTIVITY

Differentiating between the distribution of medications in the body

The principles of pharmacokinetics and pharmacodynamics are different for different drugs. With IV medications, L and A from LADME are not used; instead, the relevant phases are DME – distribution, metabolism and excretion.

Table 2.3 gives an example of the phases for phenytoin between the following medications by using information searching skills on the Internet.

TABLE 2.3 Learning pharmacokinetics

Generic (chemical) name	Common trade names in Australia	Common uses	Recommended modes of administration	Distribution and metabolism	Excretion
phenytoin	Dilantin	epilepsy	oral, parenteral (IV only)	distributed and metabolised by liver	mostly via bile and urine

Using searching skills on the Internet, find the trade name, common uses, modes of administration, distribution and metabolism, and excretion for:

1 metoclopramide
2 dexamethasone (commonly used to reduce acute or long-term inflammation).

CASE STUDY

Pharmacodynamics and pharmacokinetics

Chelsey is an EN. She works in a busy surgical ward of a small private hospital. Dr Fontaine usually prescribes cephazolin 1 g 6 hourly, IV as a prophylactic antibiotic for orthopaedic cases. Chelsey often looks after patients during the routine administration of IV cephazolin. She follows the policy guidelines at her hospital about the administration of IV medications for ENs.

One day, there is no cephazolin left in the ward. Chelsey reports this to the registered nurse (RN). The RN rings Dr Fontaine and the hospital manager. The manager says the supply of cephazolin IV is not available until tomorrow. Dr Fontaine rings back and says to the RN 'not to worry … just give the patients IV Amoxil (amoxycillin), 1 g 6 hourly IV.'

Think about this scenario and discuss with your fellow students and trainer. After discussion and using your information searching skills, answer the following questions:

1 Why would the medical prescriber have chosen amoxycillin? What is similar between cephalexin and amoxycillin?

2 What are the various trade names for amoxycillin?

3 Would it be excreted from the body in the same way as cephalexin?

4 If there was an older person with limited renal function, what might be some of the issues with these antibiotics?

IV medications and incompatibilities

Incompatibility is an unwelcome reaction that can occur with IV medications. This can happen when the drug is mixed with a solution, the container that holds the drug or another drug. Two types of incompatibilities associated with IV administration are physical and chemical. (Josephson 2006; Royal College of Nursing 2010)

A drug interaction is some type of change in a drug's ability to work due to the influence of another substance. This substance can

 All verbal medication orders require documentation and verification. Legislation across the various state and territory jurisdictions require that a verbal order is followed up in writing within 24 hours.

be another drug, a chemical substance or a nutritional substance. This results in a situation where the solution is no longer best for the patient. (Josephson 2006; Nemec, Kopelent-Frank & Grief 2008; Royal College of Nursing 2010)

The main difference between incompatibility and interaction is that a drug interaction happens inside the body and is not visible to the observer, whereas a drug incompatibility occurs inside the fluid that is in the IV bag or infusion line and this is often able to be seen by the observer. (Westabrook et al. 2011)

Figure 2.1 shows precipitation due to incompatibility between substances. For example, diazepam as an IV drug does not combine well with any other medication.

Source: Lesley Scheelings

FIGURE 2.1 Precipitation of incompatible substances

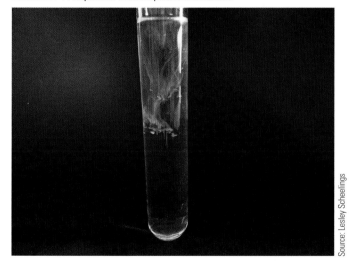

Precipitation occurs when solids develop out of any type of substance that has been mixed in a liquid solution – *this is a potentially dangerous situation.*

Any drug that precipitates when mixed with any liquid, including the IV fluid, *must* be withheld and you *must* notify the RN and/or prescribing medical practitioner.

There are many drug-related incompatibilities. These are recorded and kept up to date in Australia within the *Australian Injectable Drugs Handbook* (2014). There is a copy of this handbook in most wards or areas where IV medications are mixed and stored for usage. The information in this area is complex and ever-changing.

FNE Most solutions incompatible with plastic are provided in glass containers. See further detail in pages 532–42 of *Foundations of Nursing*.

TIP BOX

Double check

It is essential to check the *Australian Injectable Drugs Handbook* (2014) before administering an IV medication into an existing or any other IV line. It is essential to keep up to date with the latest information. This includes checking if you have the latest version of the book available or if you need to check for the latest information online.

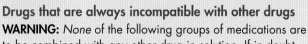

TIP BOX

Drugs that are always incompatible with other drugs

WARNING: *None* of the following groups of medications are to be combined with any other drug in solution. If in doubt, always question and ask the RN or prescribing medical practitioner:

- aminoglycosides
- chlordiazepoxide
- digitalis glycosides
- pentobarbital
- phenytoin
- secobarbital
- sodium bicarbonate
- theophylline derivatives.

 It is your legal and ethical duty to report and record any concerns about medication compatibility, regardless of the experience or seniority of the colleagues working with you.

Toxicology

Toxicology, very broadly, is defined as the study of the negative effects of chemical, physical or biological agents on living organisms and the biosphere, including the prevention and treatment of any adverse effects. (Society of Toxicology 2005)

Therefore, because medications are 'controlled poisons', the possible toxicology of medications in patients/clients needs to be considered. Medical toxicology can help you learn about and be familiar with the assessment and treatment of:

- acute or chronic poisoning
- adverse drug reactions (ADRs)
- overdoses
- envenomation
- substance abuse
- other chemical exposures.

Although it might sound odd, it is very important to remember that *medications are poisons*. Careful, professional control over the dose and administration of medications keeps their use therapeutic instead of poisonous. Government regulations around medications hint to this with their titles such as the Health, Drugs and Poisons Regulation (1996) in Queensland and the Poisons and Therapeutic Goods Regulation (2008) in New South Wales.

Figure 2.2 illustrates what can be called 'the therapeutic range' for blood levels of medication. Safe and effective administration and monitoring of medications involves keeping medication blood levels in the therapeutic range. This is so they can be the most effective – not too high to be *poisonous* – but not too low to be *ineffective* and possibly (in the case of antibiotics) a situation which increases the likelihood of antibiotic resistance developing.

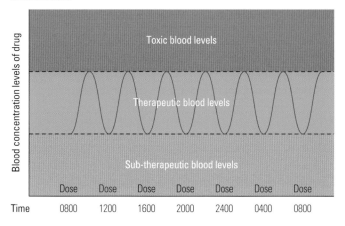

Note in **Figure 2.2** that the timing of the administration of the medication is *essential* to maintain the therapeutic range of blood levels of any medication. This is particularly important with IV medications where there is a faster rise in the blood levels and a subsequent faster fall.

CASE STUDY

Toxicology in daily nursing practice

Mavis is 84 years old. She has good health and has been on the following medications for years:

- digoxin (Lanoxin) 0.0625 mg IV mane
- frusemide (Lasix) 40 mg IV mane
- fish oil 1000 mg tablet mane.

You have assisted her with these medications for the past two years. At handover you hear that Mavis has been confused. She is also not eating as well as usual. She usually has a very good appetite. Her daughter visits with the great grandchildren. She usually loves their visits. Her daughter tells you she is concerned about her mum. She says she is 'not herself'. You document this and report this to the RN. Mavis is due to be weighed this week. You look back over her weights and note that she was 78 kg on her admission to the facility four years ago and is now 62 kg.

The RN rings the GP with the information you provided. The GP orders blood tests for Mavis. Two days later the blood tests return. Mavis is still quite confused and 'off' her food. The GP decreases Mavis's digoxin and says that it is likely that Mavis has been suffering with digitalis toxicity.

1 What may have contributed to Mavis becoming 'toxic' from digitalis after all these years?

2 How has careful collection and recording of information assisted in this early recognition and medical intervention to assist Mavis?

3 Sometimes digoxin (Lanoxin) is prescribed in micrograms instead of mg? How could this contribute to an increased risk of overdose of medication? Show your calculation of the difference.

4 If the digitalis was 'toxic', why has the GP left her on this medication?

5 Was this situation an example of acute or chronic poisoning?

 Medication safety is so important that it is one of the national safety and quality standards. See page 114 of *Foundations of Nursing*.

Factors influencing IV medication actions

Medication safety is a worldwide priority. (Australian Commission on Safety and Quality in Health Care 2014a) There are many factors that influence medication actions, including when using IV medications. These include:

- contraindications
- precautions
- ADRs
- allergy and anaphylaxis.

Contraindications and precautions

Generally contraindications and precautions will be the same for a medication given IV as via any other route. However, there are certain aspects of giving a medication via the IV route that differ.

For example, there is the need to consider the irritation that may occur to the vein or surrounding tissues from the medication being infused outside the vein and into the tissues. This creates local inflammation which is sometimes called 'tissuing'. Irritation should be checked for when monitoring IV antibiotic medications. Because of the nature of some of these medications, they can cause tissue damage to the flesh around the IV site if the medication goes into the tissues. Careful observation for this is essential.

Your job is to look for and report and record any symptoms of phlebitis. This shows as increasing pain at site of insertion of the IV, redness, swelling and heat around the IV insertion site. Phlebitis is further discussed in Chapter 5.

Your skill in information literacy (as discussed in Chapter 1) will be your key once again. Accessing the *Australian Injectable Drugs Handbook* (2014) should provide you with important pieces of information about IV medications. This will guide you in ensuring safety in administration via the recognition of side effects and precautions as well as the prevention of use under any contraindications. The Australian Commission on Safety and Quality in Health Care (2014b) is focusing on medication safety as a priority area. The website referred to in the reference list will provide you with further information about medication safety, focusing on systematic ways to make the administration of medications safer.

Another unit in your Enrolled Nursing Course – 'Administer and monitor medications in the work environment' – provides essential information for you with respect to these aspects of IV medications. (Department of Education and Training 2014)

Adverse drug reactions

Adverse drug reactions (ADRs) are much more common than **anaphylaxis**. An anaphylactic reaction is one type of ADR. There are many others.

Figure 2.3 illustrates the relationship between ADRs and anaphylactic events. The blue area in the oval represents all ADRs. The pink area represents anaphylaxis. These two areas are related but not exactly the same.

ADRs can be defined as anything from a full-blown anaphylactic event to minor common side effects. (Smith 2013)

FIGURE 2.3 The relationship of adverse drug reactions to anaphylactic events

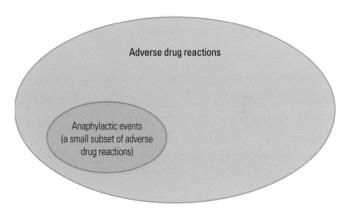

There has been a nationwide effort put into place to measure and analyse ADRs. Because of this, the Therapeutic Good Administration (TGA), which regulates medications in Australia, is eager to collect all available information about ADRs.

This reporting is usually completed by the prescribing medical practitioner. However, as an EN you will be guided by your local policies and procedures. Should you be required to report, search for TGA reporting on the Internet, which will bring up the TGA website with their reporting procedures (Department of Health Therapeutic Goods Administration 2014). The TGA website link listed in the reference list provides more information for further reading. Due to this wide range of reactions, **Table 2.4** is offered as a guide to documentation of ADRs.

TABLE 2.4 Guide to documentation of adverse drug reactions

Documentation detail	Reason for documentation
Generic and trade name of drug associated with adverse drug reaction	Trade name relevant – different medication fillers or diluents may be involved in the reaction – but this is rare
Dose, frequency and route of drug	ADRs and intolerance reactions may be dose-related
Timing of onset and offset of reaction in relation to commencement and cessation of drug	To assess likelihood of cause
Description of the reaction type (e.g. rash, behaviour change, pain)	Allows continuity of assessment
Reaction severity, management required (e.g. additional medications, hospitalisation)	May determine level of future contraindication
Original indication for use of drug (e.g. infection)	Could this have caused the reaction rather than the medication?
Cofactors (e.g. fever, other simultaneous medications)	The reaction may have been caused by an interaction between cofactors and the drug in question

Smith (2013)

FNE For more information on drug interactions, side effects and adverse reactions, see page 513 of *Foundations of Nursing*.

Allergy and anaphylaxis

Anaphylaxis is a serious, rapid-onset allergic reaction that may cause death. Severe anaphylaxis is characterised by life-threatening upper airway obstruction, bronchospasm and/or hypotension.

Common symptom areas include:

- skin (e.g. rash or hives)
- gastrointestinal tract (e.g. abdominal pain, vomiting)
- neurological (e.g. dizziness or collapse)
- respiratory (e.g. chest tightness, cough, wheeze, cyanosis)
- cardiovascular (e.g. hypotension, cardiac arrest).

Although skin rashes and hives are common, 20 per cent of anaphylaxis cases do not have any skin symptoms.

TIP BOX

Emergency management **of anaphylaxis**

- Immediately **STOP** what appears to be the causative agent. If IV is running with a medication, **STOP** this but keep the IV *in situ*.
- **Call** for assistance.

Administer **high flow oxygen** and provide **airway support** as required.

- Set up for further IV access as required – wide-bore access may be needed.
- **Prepare** for administration of IM or IV adrenaline.
- Place the patient in the **supine or recovery position** and elevate legs as tolerated.

Adapted from Brown, Mullins and Gold (2006)

SUMMARY

Within this chapter the following concepts and issues related to IV medication have been covered:

- Pharmacodynamics and pharmacokinetics are defined as what the drug does to the body and what the body does to the drug. These concepts assist in maintaining safe and effective blood levels of medications.
- Incompatibilities and drug interactions are different but equally important concepts to consider, act upon and report about in your daily nursing practice. This helps the EN to understand some of the hazards relating to IV medication administration and monitoring.

- Toxicology is the study of toxic substances. Medications are controlled toxic substances and need to be administered and monitored with caution and respect for potential problems. Your careful monitoring and administration is part of the control of these toxic substances.
- Contraindications, precautions, side effects and other occurrences such as anaphylactic and ADRs are important considerations to keep in mind during your daily nursing practice with medications in general, but even more acutely with IV medications.

REVIEW QUESTIONS

1 If you trace the route of a medication given IV from the blood vessel where it is administered to the site where it is meant to be effective and then out of the body, which body organs might be involved? How would the blood levels be affected by reduced capacity of the liver or kidney from illness or ageing?

2 In a situation where you suspect there may be a drug incompatibility or interaction, what is the *best* first action on the part of the EN (after stopping the medication)?

3 What are some of the physiological changes with ageing that contribute to the rule of 'start low and go slow' in administration and monitoring of IV medications in older people?

4 Some people will be ordered medications via an IV route. Others will be given the same medication via the oral route. Outline the difference in blood concentrations of the drug between IV and oral medication administration. How does this make IV medications potentially more dangerous?

3 PREPARING FOR AND RECORDING THE DELIVERY OF IV MEDICATIONS

LEARNING OBJECTIVES

After completing this chapter, you will be able to:

- accurately record and report relevant information relating to IV medications
- use appropriate terminology for documentation to ensure safe and effective delivery of IV medications
- prepare for and safely administer IV medications, including workplace health and safety considerations.

Introduction

This chapter will assist you to prepare for and administer IV medications. Record keeping and documentation are very important activities when administering IV medications and these are covered in this chapter. Monitoring these medications continues throughout the time they are being given. Careful attention to detail using the skills outlined here will maintain therapeutic levels of medications in the patient's bloodstream. This contributes to the safety, recovery and wellbeing of the patient.

Accurately recording and reporting relevant information

The reporting and recording of information relating to IV medications follows the same principles of documentation as covered elsewhere in the Enrolled Nursing Course. Check the units 'Apply effective communication skills in nursing practice', 'Implement and evaluate a plan of nursing care' and 'Apply legal and ethical parameters to nursing practice'. (Department of Education and Training 2014)

In order to be effective, documentation must be all of the following:

- *complete* – documentation should include objective information. Subjective information from the patient or families should be shown in quotation marks
- *accurate* – entries to documentation must be legible and easy to read with correct spelling. This is particularly important when using numbers, medical terminology and accepted abbreviations. The writing of a specific measurement provides better accuracy (e.g. he drank 300 mL of water)
- *concise* – documentation should be complete enough to give a picture of what is happening without being excessively wordy

- *factual* – you should describe the information about exactly what you see, hear, smell or feel. Do not infer cause or actions without supporting data. Vague terms such as 'appears', 'seems' or 'apparently' are not accurate. State the facts only, as you see them at the time
- *timely* – document date and time of each recording and using the 24-hour clock. Do not do any recording in advance
- *organised* – the patient's name and identifying information should be on each page. Information should be in a time sequence as much as possible and in black ink to facilitate any copying that may be required in the future (see **Figure 3.1**)
- *prudent* and *confidential* – consider that the medical record is a legal document. What is happening today may be called for evidence in court (or used to assist the patient's care) many years from now. Confidentiality is your professional duty.

Jefferies et al. (2012); Teytelman (2002)

 For further information relating to documentation skills, see Part 2 of *Essential Clinical Skills* 3rd edn (pages 45–8).

Standards for documentation

The principles of safe and effective documentation in nursing practice as outlined by the ANMC's (Australian Nursing and Midwifery Council) National Competency Standards for the Enrolled Nurse (2002) are shown on page 26.

 For more information about the principles of effective documentation, see pages 196–200 of *Foundations of Nursing*.

FIGURE 3.1 **Example of documentation of information**

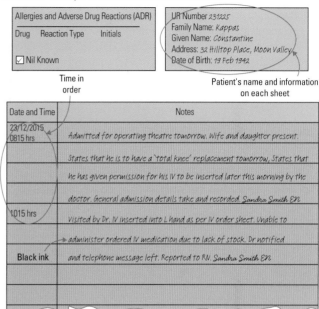

 Medical records are legal documents.

Competency element 7.3: Ensures communication, reporting and documentation are timely and accurate.

- Communicates information to individuals/groups accurately and in accordance with organisational policies regarding disclosure of information
- Clarifies written orders for nursing care with the registered nurse when unclear
- Documents nursing care in accordance with organisational policy
- Documents nursing care in a comprehensive, logical, legible, accurate, clear and concise manner, using accepted abbreviations and terminologies when appropriate
- Demonstrates awareness of legal requirements governing written documentation and consults with the registered nurse to ensure these requirements are met

Australian Nursing and Midwifery Council (2002, p. 7)

ACTIVITY

Linking the national standards to practice

For each of the listed five competencies above, describe a brief nursing action where you would be demonstrating your competence. There is one example already given for each. Write another example for each.

1 Communicates information to individuals/groups accurately and in accordance with organisational policies regarding disclosure of information.
   Example: Professionally discusses the concerns about the patient's IV with the family, explaining the need for IV medications.

2 Clarifies written orders for nursing care with the registered nurse when unclear.
   Example: Unsure of the dose as the writing of the medication order is unclear. Checks with RN.

3 Documents nursing care in accordance with organisational policy.

Example: Uses consistent initials for signature. Adds this in each area where initials are requested on documents or where hospital policy dictates.

4 Documents nursing care in a comprehensive, logical, legible, accurate, clear and concise manner, using accepted abbreviations and terminologies when appropriate.
   Example: Practises writing nursing notes about any unusual or new situation on scrap paper and checks with RN before writing in record when unsure.

5 Demonstrates awareness of legal requirements governing written documentation and consults with the registered nurse to ensure these requirements are met.
   Example: Writes exact date and time when making notes about pain and swelling at IV insertion site. Reports verbally to RN and advises of documentation.

Commonly accepted terms and abbreviations

Many of the commonly accepted documentation terms and abbreviations used in IV medications are the same as the ones used with any medications. There is a comprehensive list of acceptable general Australian abbreviations that you can access. It is provided by the Australian Commission on Safety and Quality in Health Care. (Arcus et al. 2011) Table 3.1 provides a sample of commonly used abbreviations with IV medications; the Australian Commission on Safety and Quality in Health Care provides a more extensive list, covering most known situations associated with medications. This includes a national guideline that is under development and will be available from the Commission with regard to consistent displays of medication information in an electronic format.

 Using approved abbreviations and symbols is a legal requirement in documentation.

ACTIVITY

Using abbreviations

Search for and find the document above by the Australian Commission on Safety and Quality in Health Care (Arcus et al. 2011). Go to 'Table 2: Acceptable Terms and Abbreviations'. Then do the following:

1 Copy the commonly used abbreviations and their related meaning from Table 3.1 in this chapter.

2 Add any additional definitions you might find during the course of your clinical practice in IV administration.

3 In a group, discuss when you or a doctor might use these abbreviations.

TABLE 3.1 Sample of commonly used abbreviations in the delivery of IV medications

Intended meaning	Acceptable terms or abbreviations	Category of abbreviation
every 4 hours; every 4 hrs	4 hourly	Dose frequency or timing
every 6 hours; every 6 hrs	6 hourly	Dose frequency or timing
when required	prn	Dose frequency or timing
immediately	stat	Dose frequency or timing
intravenous	IV	Route of administration
intravenous injection	IV inj	Route of administration
gram(s)	g	Units of measure
milligram(s)	mg	Units of measure
millilitre(s)	mL	Units of measure
litre(s)	L	Units of measure
injection	inj	Dose forms
powder	powder	Dose forms
patient controlled analgesia	PCA	Dose forms

Arcus et al. (2011). 'Recommendations for Terminology, Abbreviations and Symbols used in the Prescribing and Administration of Medicines'. Australian Commission on Safety and Quality in Health Care. http://www.safetyandquality.gov.au/wp-content/uploads/2012/01/32060v2.pdf

ECS For further information relating to terms and abbreviations, see Part 4 of *Essential Clinical Skills* 3rd edn (pages 103–25).

Safety is of the utmost importance when dealing with medications, especially when they are given intravenously. Error-prone abbreviations have been highlighted by the Australian Commission on Safety and Quality in Health Care. (Arcus et al. 2011) **Table 3.2** provides a sample of error-prone abbreviations associated with IV medications.

Documentation is often best learnt by practice. Read the following scenarios related to medication and IV charts and answer the questions related to the chart as practice.

TABLE 3.2 Sample of error-prone abbreviations and symbols

Error-prone abbreviation (not to be used)	Intended meaning	Why?	What should be used
IJ	injection	mistaken as intrajugular or IV	inj or injection
6/24	every six hours	mistaken as six times a day	'every 6 hours' or '6 hourly' or '6 hrly'
4/24	every four hours	mistaken as four times a day	'every 4 hours' or '4 hourly' or '4 hrly'
No leading zero before a decimal dose (e.g. 0.5 mg)	0.5 mg	mistaken as 5 mg if decimal point not seen	ensure there is a zero before a decimal point when dose is less than a whole unit
Use of trailing zero after decimal point (e.g. 1.0 mg)	1 mg	mistaken as 10 mg if decimal point not seen	ensure there is no trailing zero for doses in whole numbers

Arcus et al. (2011). 'Recommendations for Terminology, Abbreviations and Symbols used in the Prescribing and Administration of Medicines'. Australian Commission on Safety and Quality in Health Care. http://www.safetyandquality.gov.au/wp-content/uploads/2012/01/32060v2.pdf

IV fluid orders

Mavis McCarthy is an 80-year-old woman requiring intravenous fluids for dehydration. She is ordered the intravenous fluids shown on the medication chart in **Figure 3.2**.

1 Where would you sign for this bag of IV fluid?

2 Who would be 'nurse' and who would be 'checker'?

FIGURE 3.2 Mavis McCarthy IV fluid medication order

Intravenous fluid treatment				Mavis McCarthy 42 Green Drive, Nungarin DOB 19.02.1935				Birthdate	

Date	Start time	Bot. no.	Volume	Type of fluid	Additives	Rate	Doctor's signature/ name	Signatures 1 Nurse 2 Checker
02.08.2015	Stat	1	1 litre	0.9% normal saline	NIL	4 hourly	JG Ganesha	

CASE STUDY

Fluid balance charts

Marco Lavanza is a man admitted to hospital requiring intravenous fluids while fasting for an operation. He is ordered the intravenous fluids shown on the chart in Figure 3.3.

Marco (and most patients) must have a fluid balance chart while on an IV. Look at the fluid balance chart in Figure 3.4. Where would you write the following information:

1 When the IV bag of 1000 mL was started?
2 When Marco used the urine bottle and you measured 420 mL as you emptied it?
3 When he vomited and you measured 100 mL as you emptied it?

FIGURE 3.3 Intravenous fluid treatment: medication order

Intravenous fluid treatment				Marco Lavanza 35 Brolga Lane, Seaview DOB 13.06.1990			Birthdate		

Date	Start time	Bot. no.	Volume	Type of fluid	Additives	Rate	Doctor's signature/ name	Signatures 1 Nurse 2 Checker
26.05.2015	Stat	1	1 litre	Hartmanns	NIL	12 hourly	JC Connor	

FIGURE 3.4 Fluid balance chart

Fluid Balance Chart (Adult)

NHS

Name:	Marco Lavanza
Address	35 Brolga Lane, Seaview
DOB:	13.06.1990
CRN/ Hospital No:	UR12345

Ward: .... 6B .... Consultant: ...... Michael Hendricks .... Patient's weight: .... 92 kg ....

Date: .... 26.05.2015 .... Refer to Guidelines if chart is predominantly used for input only (e.g. Rehab)

Time	Intake: mL						Output: mL						
	Oral	IV (1)	IV (2)	Other		Running Total	Urine*	NG	Other (chest drain, etc)			Running Total	Initials
06.00													
07.00													
08.00													
09.00													
10.00													
11.00													
12.00													

FNE For more detailed information on fluid, electrolyte and acid–base balance, see Chapter 21 of *Foundations of Nursing* (pages 474–505).

Preparing for the administration of IV medications

Most commonly, IV medications are administered via a **peripheral line**. This means that the IV cannula is inserted into a vein that is usually in part of the body away from the centre, such as the arm or leg.

Preparing to start the IV line

Planning the required equipment in advance saves time and reduces errors. You will need:

- the medical order
- the bag (occasionally, bottle) of IV fluid as per order (check that the order and the fluid type match)
- IV tubing to match situation (this is for a simple gravity-fed IV without any infusion pump).

There are many types of IV tubing. The standard one will be shown here that produces 20 drops per mL in the drip chamber.

There are other types of tubing (which can come with the giving set attached):

- *Microdrip tubing* is a type of IV giving set with tubing that delivers 60 drops per mL of IV fluid. This is most commonly used in paediatric and high acuity care situations.
- *Extension tubing* is a piece of tubing which is used to connect the cannula, which has been inserted into the vein, to the IV line. This tubing can have a narrower lumen. It needs to be changed regularly according to local hospital policy.
- *Specific tubing to suit particular infusion pumps* is produced by a manufacturer of infusion pumps, which can have its own type of

tubing. Each type of pump is to be used with the specific tubing for the pump as outlined in the specifications for the pump.

Most tubing has a roller in place to control the flow of fluid manually, in drops per minute. **Figure 3.5** show a commonly used roller on a standard peripheral line.

 For further information relating to preparation, see Part 7.2 'Intravenous therapy (IVT) – assisting with establishment' of *Essential Clinical Skills* 3rd edn (pages 213–17).

FIGURE 3.5 **A manual roller used to control the drops per minute**

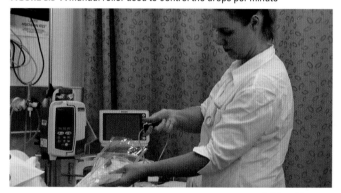

Tollefson video source

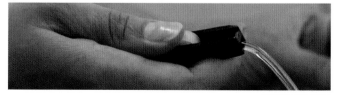

Tollefson video source

You may need to gather a range of IV cannula types and sizes as well as a dressing pack when you are assisting a medical officer or suitably skilled RN to cannulate the patient.

 Mostly IVs are started by medical officers but some RNs have certification. Check your local policies.

As much as possible, the 'set up' should be completed *well before* the person arrives to do the cannulation (see **Figure 3.6**).

Depending on local policies, you may need a separate medical order for each bag of fluid. Details of exact requirements depend on how the fluid order was written by the medical practitioner.

FIGURE 3.6 'Set up' for cannulation

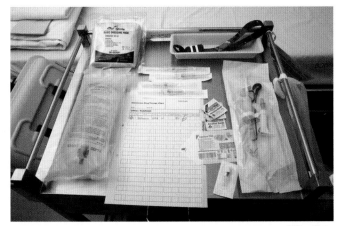

© Doug Steley

IV fluid bags come with an outer covering bag. *Do not* use a bag of IV fluid that has had the outer bag removed, as this increases the risk of something having been added to the bag. Do these other checks at this time:

- Check the written medical order against what is written on the bag.
- Check the expiry date of the fluid – if it is after this date, do not use the fluid.
- Check the bag for leakage.
- Check for 'floaties' in the bag, in case there has been some precipitation (which happens rarely).

Priming the IV line

One of the activities related to your preparation is to **prime the IV line**. Priming a line means that you are ensuring the fluid has *half-filled the drip chamber* and *fully-filled the tubing* with no air. The half-filled drip chamber is to see and count the drops in the chamber.

There are problems with having air in the IV tubing. These are:

- **air embolism**, which is the most lethal (but rare) and, in some cases, can be fatal
- decreased accuracy in measurement of fluids
- air-locks, which can stop the fluids from moving freely through the tubing.

Priming the IV line

1 Use **aseptic non-touch technique (ANTT)** (outlined in Chapter 5, page 67) to remove the cover on the bottom of the bag of IV fluid and the top of the tubing with the trocar. Ensure the

manual roller is closed on the tubing. There is a variety of styles of doing this – most of them work. You can leave the roller further down the tubing, but putting it near the drip chamber offers a bit more control for the beginner.

2   After washing your hands, insert the piercing end of the tubing into the IV bag (sometimes called 'spiking' the bag), using a firm grip on the bag and the IV tubing. **Figure 3.7** shows the use of a firm pushing and twisting motion with both hands. This will help to get the trocar in place firmly and correctly.

3   Now squeeze the drip chamber to fill it half way, as illustrated in **Figure 3.8**. Be sure not to overfill. Leave space so the drops can be counted as they fall from the bag. Keep roller closed on tubing during this time.

FIGURE 3.7 **Inserting the trocar**

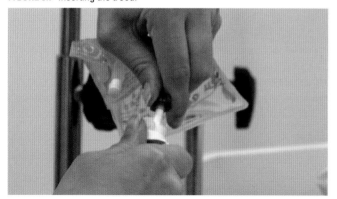

Tollefson video source

FIGURE 3.8 **Squeezing the drip chamber**

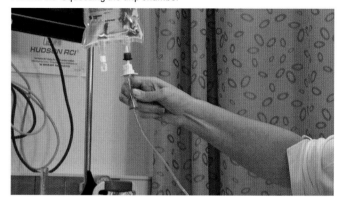

Tollefson video source

4   Once you are certain that the drip chamber is about half full, *slowly* release the roller on the tubing, as illustrated in **Figure 3.9**. This will cause fluid to run and drops to come into the chamber.

5   Run this until the fluid reaches the end of the tubing. Keep the end of the tubing sterile using ANTT. Take the cap off to connect it to the IV cannula that has been inserted into the patient's vein (see **Figure 3.10**).

6   Now adjust the roller while counting the drops to ensure the line is running and the rate is according to the medical order.

FIGURE 3.9 Releasing the roller

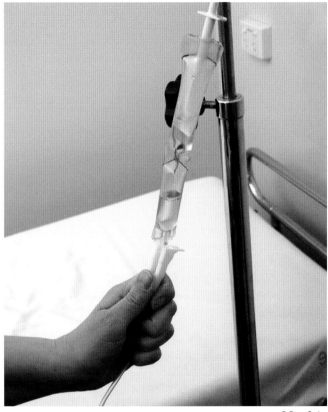

© Doug Steley

FIGURE 3.10 Connecting the tubing

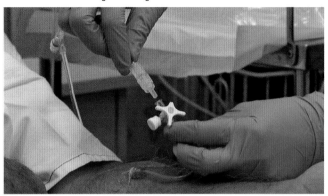

Tollefson video source

Clean up any rubbish, using the principles of infection control and occupational health and safety as outlined in other units in your Enrolled Nursing Course. (Department of Education and Training 2014) Tidy up the area where you have been working. Document the following information about the IV commencement:

- Date
- Time
- Vessel used and/or limb location
- Type of fluid and amounts on both IV fluid orders and fluid balance chart.

 For more detailed information on fluid balance (sometimes called intake and output), see Chapter 21 of *Foundations of Nursing* (pages 474–505).

Preparing for injecting medications into IV lines

Preparation for giving IV medications is similar to the administration of any medication as outlined in your unit on the administration of medication. (Department of Education and Training 2014) There are extra steps that are required to prepare the medication for IV administration (as follows).

The first step is to check for accuracy of details *three* times: once when preparing, once when mixing and again at the bedside.

One of the first checks is guided by the '5 rights'.

When you are doing your Enrolled Nursing Course you learn about the essential '5 rights' of medication administration during your medication unit (Department of Education and Training 2014):

- Right patient
- Right time
- Right dose
- Right drug
- Right route.

There is some variation between workplaces and various states and territories. Each location may add some or all of the following important rights to their list of 'rights':

- Right to refuse
- Right expiry date
- Right documentation
- Right knowledge of any allergies
- Right to know information about the drug.

There are several ways that IV medications are available for injection. Powders are common. They require reconstitution with sterile water or normal saline, depending on recommendations found in the most up-to-date *Australian Injectable Drugs Handbook* (SHPA 2014). An up-to-date version of this book should be available when IV drugs are being administered.

How to reconstitute powdered IV medication

1   To begin, gather the supplies required to reconstitute the powdered IV medication. This includes:
    - the medication ordered (checked with 5 'rights' – or the local number required)
    - the diluent (usually normal saline or water)
    - a syringe (size depends on amount of diluent required)
    - an 18-gauge needle
    - a sharps container
    - a general rubbish container
    - alcohol wipes.

    Use the manufacturer's recommendations for amount of fluid (diluent) for reconstitution to use; this should be written on the vial and in the *Australian Injectable Drugs Handbook* (2014). **WARNING**: Check that the diluent actually has 'Water for Injection' or 'Normal Saline for Injection' on the tube. Fatal errors have been made by mixing the medication with other fluids that look similar.

2   Gather supplies and re-check that the particulars of the order match the equipment gathered, the patient's details, the time required and all other details.

3   Open the syringe from its package and loosen.

4   Twist off the top of the fluid (diluent) that most often comes in plastic flexible bottles (after checking accuracy on side of ampoule) (see **Figure 3.11**).

5 Attach a syringe (without a needle) to fluid and draw back required amount.

6 Open bottom of needle case (see **Figure 3.12**) and attach the 18-gauge needle to syringe (see **Figure 3.13**).

7 Wipe top of powder vial with alcohol wipe in the rare event that it does not come with a cap in place, or according to local policy.

8 Insert needle into the rubber bung on the powder vial.

9 Inject enough fluid to dilute the powder, depending on manufacturer's instructions and how the IV medication is to be administered.

10 Gently move the vial to dissolve the medication into solution.

FIGURE 3.11 Checking accuracy of diluent on the side of the ampoule

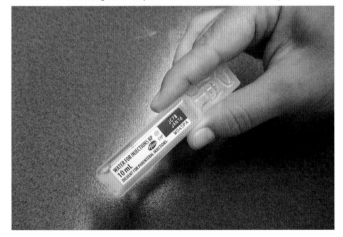

FIGURE 3.12 Opening needle case

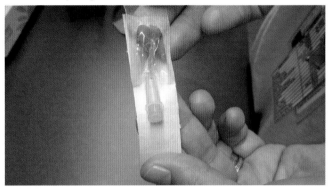

FIGURE 3.13 Attaching 18-gauge needle

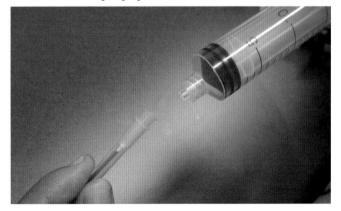

11   Draw the medication back up into the syringe.

12   Some local policies advocate writing on the syringe – the name of drug and diluent – for further safety.

Your IV medication is now prepared and ready to be given.

Now re-check the medication against the medical order before giving to the patient so you know you have the 5 rights covered (see earlier in this section).

When actually injecting the IV bolus, it is important to:

- inject slowly over at least three minutes, unless otherwise indicated in manufacturer's instructions
- always check local policies and procedures and manufacturer's recommendations

- maintain ANTT
- watch the patient's veins for any signs of inflammation – redness, swelling, increasing pain, increased heat.

 Consider your legal and ethical duty of care.

TIP BOX

Safely injecting IV boluses

Injecting too fast into a vein can cause collapse of the vein, irritation of the tissues and, sometimes, phlebitis.

CASE STUDY

Taking verbal orders

Elisha is an EN who has passed all of her competency assessments for IV medications. She works in theatre across the various areas as a 'casual' – in the hope that she may get a permanent role. As her patient was wheeled into the recovery area, a doctor says, 'Oh, I forgot to give the IV ceftriaxone – can you give in recovery?'

Elisha asks the doctor to write this up on the patient's medication chart in the appropriate place. She checks the ceftriaxone with the RN and dilutes it according to local policies and procedures and manufacturer's instructions. The RN says to Elisha, 'Hurry up, we have to get this guy out of here, there

are more patients coming' … as Elisha is slowly injecting this IV antibiotic into the vein to prevent phlebitis. Consider the following questions for yourself and discuss with your colleagues as to what might be the best course of action:

1   What would be Elisha's most appropriate response to the RN's request?

2   How can she diplomatically handle this situation while saving the patient's veins?

 Consider Elisha's scenario carefully; it has both legal and ethical issues for discussion.

Within this chapter the following concepts and issues related to IV medication have been covered:

- It is important to accurately report and record any activity associated with IV medications. Following the principles of clear and accurate documentation are necessary.
- Accurate and consistent terminology prevents errors. Checking about the meaning of terminology or abbreviations is never wrong and will prevent errors and mistakes.
- Preparation is essential for safe administration of IV medications. This includes establishing the IV line, preparation of the medication and checking the medication with colleagues.
- Because working with IV medications means the use of sharps and working near bodily fluids, it is *essential* to follow the principles of infection control and workplace health and safety as outlined in your Enrolled Nursing Course units related to these topics.

REVIEW QUESTIONS

1 List the steps of effective documentation. Write an example related to the administration of IV medications.
2 Outline five abbreviations commonly used in relation to IV medications that are nationally provided by the Australian Commission on Safety and Quality in Health Care.
3 Write an example of how you would measure how much fluid needs to be written on the fluid balance chart when a patient has an IV and has had a cup of tea.
4 Why is it absolutely essential to use ANTT when preparing for the insertion of an IV line?
5 Whose responsibility is it to maintain asepsis?
6 What does it mean to prime an IV line during preparation for the commencement of IV fluids?
7 How would you find out how to prepare a powdered medication for IV injection that you have never seen before?
8 How often should you check your IV medications for accuracy?
9 Why are IV medications more risky to the patient than tablets or capsules given orally?

4 MAJOR IV MEDICATION GROUPS

LEARNING OBJECTIVES

After completing this chapter, you will be able to:
- describe the different classes of IV medication groups
- list at least one or two IV medications within the following groups – antibiotics; antifungal, antiviral and antiprotozoal agents; cardiovascular agents; CNS agents; drugs affecting electrolyte and water balance; gastrointestinal agents; haematological agents; hormones and synthetic substances; and vitamins and minerals
- discuss the actions, adverse reactions and nursing management required for each of the medications described.

Introduction

Understanding the major IV medication groups is necessary so that the EN can:
- identify certain classes of IV medications that produce particular therapeutic responses in the body
- understand why they are selected to treat certain clinical conditions
- know why they are reconstituted or added to particular infusions
- understand the monitoring required of patients
- know the pharmacological actions and responses as a result of administering IV medications.

IV medication administration is governed by local policy. You must become familiar with what is allowed from a direct supervision perspective and what is purely maintenance of an IV medication administration.

This chapter briefly discusses some IV medications in each class; to gain a more in-depth understanding, refer to *Pharmacology in Nursing: Australia and New Zealand* (Broyles et al. 2013).

Antibiotics

The largest category of commonly used IV medications is **antibiotics**. Antibiotics destroy bacterial organisms and can be classified into two different groups based on their mechanism of action: bactericidal agents and bacteriostatic agents. Bactericidal agents kill the bacteria and are used for the treatment of serious infections or when the patient has a compromised immune system. Bacteriostatic agents retard the growth of the bacteria and work in conjunction with the patient's immune system to destroy and remove the bacteria.

Antibiotics can also be described according to their spectrum:

- *Narrow-spectrum antibiotics* target Gram-negative or Gram-positive bacteria. They are effective agents when the bacteria has been identified as the cause of the infection and is susceptible to the action of the particular narrow-spectrum antibiotic. These agents are somewhat safer than broad-spectrum antibiotics as they do not interfere with the normal bacterial flora of the body. An example of a narrow-spectrum antibiotic is penicillin G (benzylpenicillin).
- *Broad-spectrum antibiotics* affect a wide range of bacteria and are useful when the identity and susceptibility of the bacteria has not been established. These agents have the ability to destroy the body's normal bacterial flora, as it targets a wide range of organisms. Examples of broad-spectrum antibiotics are carbapenems, tetracycline and ticarcillin.

Mechanism of action

Antibiotics can work to kill bacteria in three different ways. It is important to know the mechanism of action of an antibiotic to target and kill the right bacteria:

- *Bactericidal drugs* kill the bacteria directly by either inhibiting the synthesis of the cell wall or by interfering with the cell membrane permeability to destroy the cell wall. Examples are beta lactams – penicillins (e.g. flucloxacillin, see **Figure 4.1**), cephalosporins (e.g. cephazolin sodium), carbapenems (e.g. meropenem, see **Figure 4.2**) – and aminoglycosides (e.g. gentamycin), quinolones (ciprofloxacin) and vancomycin (see **Figure 4.3**).

FIGURE 4.1 Flucloxacillin a beta-lactam (penicillin) is bactericidal

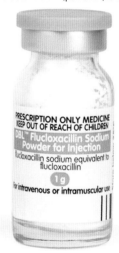

Hospira, Inc.

FIGURE 4.2 Meropenem, a carbapenem, is bactericidal

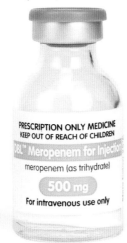

Hospira, Inc.

FIGURE 4.3 Vancomycin is bactericidal

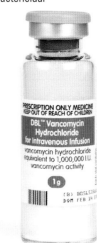

Hospira, Inc.

- *Bacteriostatic drugs* prevent the growth of the bacteria by interfering with bacterial protein production, DNA replication or bacterial cellular metabolism. They work with the immune system to remove the bacteria. Examples are the macrolides (e.g. erythromycin and clindamycin).
- Drugs that are *both* bacteriostatic and bactericidal can block or alter the growth of the bacteria as they interfere with metabolites required for normal function. Examples are

sulfonamides (trimethoprim–sulfamethoxazole) and chloramphenicol sodium succinate (Chloromycetin). (Alexander et al. 2010, pp. 263–98; Broyles et al. 2013, p. 112)

Antibacterial agents

Antibacterial agents can be classified into many categories including beta lactams (penicillins cephalosporins, carbapenems), tetracyclines, macrolides, aminoglycosides and quinolones.

Penicillins

Penicillins are important antibiotics because they are low cost, have a low toxicity and have good clinical efficacy when treating many infections.

Classification: Penicillins are bactericidal.

Action: They inhibit the synthesis of the bacterial cell wall, destroying the organism. Benzylpenicillin is an example of a narrow-spectrum penicillin (see **Figure 4.4**).

Adverse effects: These are varied with penicillins; the most common is hypersensitivity reactions. Hypersensitivity can be divided into four basic types:

- Dermatological reactions (i.e. itch, hives and/or rashes).
- Serum-like reactions are evident 6 to 10 days after the administration and are characterised by fever, malaise, hives, joint pain, muscle pain, swollen lymph nodes and an enlarged spleen. These reactions have a short life span and are gone within days or weeks after the drug has been ceased.
- Haematological reactions are related to large doses of penicillin; the reaction causes anaemia.
- Anaphylaxis is the most serious hypersensitivity, and generally occurs within the first 30 minutes of administration. Symptoms may include hypotension, arrhythmia, respiratory congestion, laryngeal oedema, nausea and diarrhoea. Anaphylaxis requires immediate emergency action to maintain a patent airway: administer adrenaline, oxygen therapy and corticosteroids. (Alexander et al. 2010, pp. 263–98)

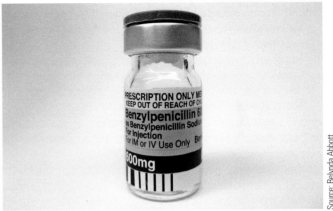

FIGURE 4.4 Benzylpenicillin is a narrow-spectrum antibiotic

Cephalosporins

Cephalosporins have a similar structure to penicillins.

Classification: Cephalosporins are bactericidal and are classified by their generation or also known as their spectrum of activity:

- First-generation cephalosporins (e.g. cephazolin and cephalexin) are active against Gram-positive bacteria (e.g. *Staphylococcus aureus* and *Staphylococcus epidermidis*) and some Gram-negative bacteria.
- Second-generation cephalosporins (e.g. cefaclor, cefoxitin and cefuroxime) have a greater Gram-negative activity and a diminished activity against Gram-positive bacteria.

- Third-generation cephalosporins (e.g. ceftazidime and ceftriaxone) are active against Gram-negative bacteria and are less effective against Gram-positive bacteria than second-generation cephalosporins.
- Fourth-generation cephalosporins (e.g. cefepime) are similar to the third-generation cephalosporins, although they have the greatest action against Gram-negative bacteria and minimal action against Gram-positive bacteria.

Action: Cephalosporins disrupt the synthesis of the bacterial cell wall, causing the wall to break down and so destroying the organism.

Adverse effects: Cephalosporin reactions can be similar to penicillin and can range from a mild rash to anaphylaxis. Therefore caution must be considered when the patient has an allergy history to penicillin. Nephrotoxicity is rare but likely to occur in patients with a history of renal impairment. (Alexander et al. 2010, pp. 263–98; Broyles et al. 2013, p. 115)

Carbapenems

Classification: Carbapenems are beta-lactam broad-spectrum antibiotics.

Action: They inhibit cell wall synthesis. They are effective against many aerobic and anaerobic bacteria. Carbapenems include imipenem and meropenem.

Adverse effects: These include gastrointestinal effects (nausea, vomiting and diarrhoea), hypersensitivity, CNS effects (seizures) and potential for cross-reactivity in patients allergic to penicillins or cephalosporins.

Tetracyclines

Classification: Tetracyclines were the first broad-spectrum antibiotic developed and are bacteriostatic.

Action: They inhibit protein synthesis within the cell. Tetracyclines include doxycycline (Vibramycin).

Adverse effects: These include gastrointestinal effects, hypersensitivity, venous irritation and photosensitivity.

Macrolides

Classification: Macrolides are mostly bacteriostatic but have some bactericidal activity when administered in high concentrations. The only IV macrolide used is erythromycin lactobionate.

Action: Erythromycin is mainly used for staphylococcal, pneumococcal and streptococcal infections, and in the treatment of Legionnaire's disease. It is metabolised in the liver. Another macrolide is azithromycin (see **Figure 4.5**), which is used to treat upper and lower respiratory tract infections.

Adverse effects: Caution must be considered when administering these drugs to patients with impaired liver function.

Aminoglycosides

Classification: Aminoglycosides are bactericidal and effective against several Gram-negative organisms.

Action: Aminoglycosides inhibit protein synthesis in the cell.

Adverse effects: These include nephrotoxicity, ototoxicity and neuromuscular-blocking action resulting in respiratory paralysis.

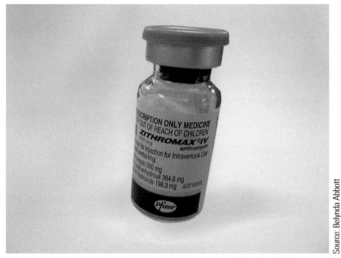

Quinolones

Classification: Quinolones are bactericidal.

Action: Quinolones inhibit an enzyme that leads to DNA fragmentation, killing the organism. They are effective against Gram-positive and Gram-negative bacteria, especially *Pseudomonas aeruginosa*. Ciprofloxacin is an example of a quinolone.

Adverse effects: These include hypersensitivity, photosensitivity, CNS reactions (insomnia, manic reactions and toxic psychosis) and tendon rupture.

Other antibiotics

Other antibiotics that do not belong to a specific classification have differing chemical structures; however, they share common properties with all antibiotics. The IV antibiotics within this group include the following.

Vancomycin

Classifcation: Vancomycin (see **Figure 4.3** on page 42) is a tricyclic glycopeptide antibiotic and is bactericidal.

Action: It works against Gram-positive bacteria, as it inhibits cell wall synthesis, cell membrane permeability and RNA synthesis. It is used in serious infections including endocarditis, septicaemia and bone, lower respiratory tract and skin infections.

Adverse effects: Vancomycin when administered intravenously is a known **vesicant** and can cause ototoxicity, nephrotoxicity and hypersensitivity reactions. It is important to administer vancomycin intermittently, diluted no more than 5 mg/mL and infused over 1–2 hours. (Gahart & Nazareno 2014, pp. 1190–4)

Clindamycin

Classification: Clindamycin is bacteriostatic and active against Gram-positive aerobic and anaerobic bacteria and some Gram-negative anaerobic bacteria.

Action: It inhibits protein synthesis in the cell. Clindamycin is chemically related to and acts like erythromycin.

Adverse effects: These include gastrointestinal effects and hypersensitivities.

Chloramphenicol

Classification: Chloramphenicol sodium succinate (Chloromycetin) is effective against Gram-positive and Gram-negative bacteria. It is predominantly bacteriostatic but may be bactericidal if used in high concentrations.

Action: It acts by inhibiting protein synthesis. It is important to administer Chloromycetin intermittently.

Adverse effects: It can cause haematological effects leading to bone marrow depression. (Gahart & Nazareno 2014, pp. 1190–4)

Sulfonamides

Classification: Sulfonamides have a broad spectrum and are usually bacteriostatic.

Action: They work by depriving the bacteria of folate required for DNA synthesis. Trimethoprim+sulfamethoxazole (cotrimoxazole) is a unique bactericidal antibiotic that combines a sulfonamide with trimethoprim to reduce bacterial resistance. This combination blocks two steps that are required by the bacteria to form folic acid.

Adverse effects: These include hypersensitivity, renal dysfunction and haematological changes. Adequate hydration and increased monitoring and observations of patients is required.

Antibiotic resistance

Antibiotic resistance is a big threat to treatment of bacterial infections.

Discuss the reasons why resistance has emerged over time and what role you have as an EN to assist with decreasing the risk of further antibiotic resistance.

Antifungal, antiviral and antiprotozoal agents

Other IV medications may be required to treat infections that are not caused by bacterial organisms but by organisms such as fungi, viruses and protozoa; these medications are antifungals agents, antiviral agents and antiprotozoal agents (see **Table 4.1**).

TABLE 4.1 Different types of IV antifungal, antiviral and antiprotozoal agents

Antifungal agents	Antiviral agents	Antiprotozoal agents
Amphotericin Fluconazole (**Figure 4.6**) Voriconazole	Aciclovir Ganciclovir	Metronidazole (Flagyl) (**Figure 4.7**)

Antifungal agents

Antifungal agents include amphotericin and the azoles.

Antifungal agents act by binding to sterols within the membrane of the fungal cell, leading to cell death. Sterols are not found within bacteria.

Adverse effects from infusion of amphotericin include headache, chills, fever, malaise, anorexia, nausea and vomiting. Similar adverse effects are related to fluconazole (see **Figure 4.6**) and voriconazole.

FIGURE 4.6 Fluconazole is an antifungal agent

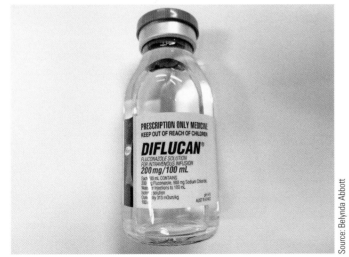

Source: Belynda Abbott

Antiviral agents

Antiviral agents inhibit the viral replication process, allowing the body's immune system to defend against the viral infection. Adverse effects include nausea, vomiting, infusion phlebitis at the site, and nephrotoxicity.

Antiprotozoal agents

An example of an antiprotozoal agent is metronidazole (see **Figure 4.7**). Intravenously it is effective in the treatment of

FIGURE 4.7 Metronidazole is an antiprotozoal agent

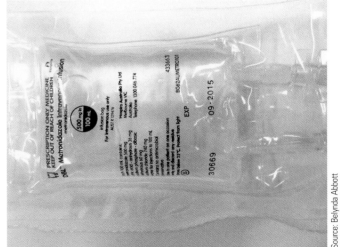

Hospira, Inc.

Source: Belynda Abbott

amoebiasis, trichomoniasis, giardiasis and infections caused by anaerobic bacteria. It interferes with the protozoal cell by inactivating its function and replication. Adverse effects of metronidazole include nausea, headaches and abdominal cramping. (Gahart & Nazareno 2014, pp. 799–802; Alexander et al. 2010, p. 279; Broyles et al. 2013, p. 143)

Cardiovascular agents

Cardiovascular agents are used for numerous actions – including cardiac strength, rate and rhythm – to counteract hypotension and control hypertension, and to improve circulation. (Alexander et al. 2010, p. 282) The IV cardiovascular agents discussed in this chapter include antihypertensives, antiarrhythmics and cardiac stimulants. An important nursing consideration with IV cardiovascular agents is that the patient must be cardiac monitored and there must be appropriate emergency equipment available at the time of administration.

Antihypertensives

'Antihypertensive' is the classification given to the class of drugs that treat hypertension (high blood pressure).

Beta blockers

Classification: Beta blockers are the antagonist of beta receptors of the sympathetic nervous system.

Action: Beta receptors are located in the heart muscle. When these are blocked by beta blockers, there is a decreased pulse rate, a decreased firing rate in the sinoatrial node and decreased myocardial muscle contractility of the heart, reducing cardiac output. Beta blockers are used to treat hypertension, cardiac dysrhythmias, angina and as a prophylactic. (Broyles et al. 2013, p. 209) The two common beta blockers that are used intravenously are propranolol and metoprolol.

Adverse effects: These include bradycardia, hypotension, insomnia, depression, constipation and hypoglycaemia.

TIP BOX

Remembering a beta blocker
An easy way to remember a beta blocker is that the generic drug name will probably end in 'lol' (e.g. metoprolol and propanolol).

Calcium channel blockers

Classification: Calcium channel blockers are also known as calcium antagonists.

Action: Calcium channel blockers prevent the movement of calcium into the cardiac and smooth muscle cells when they are stimulated, therefore decreasing contractibility and decreasing blood pressure and cardiac workload. Calcium channel blockers include IV drugs such as diltiazem, verapamil and nicardipine.

Adverse effects: These include dizziness, headache, fatigue, nausea, hepatic injury, hypotension, bradycardia, peripheral oedema and heart block. (Broyles et al. 2013, p. 334)

Vasodilators

Classification: Vasodilators re antihypertensives that are classified in accordance with their site or mechanism of action.

Action: Vasodilators act on vascular smooth muscle within either the arterial or venous system to relax the muscle; this results in vasodilation and decreased blood pressure. Examples of IV vasodilators are diazoxide, hydralazine and nitroprusside.

Adverse effects: These include dizziness, anxiety, headache, reflex tachycardia, congestive heart failure, chest pain, oedema, skin rash, hypotension, nausea and vomiting. Nitroglycerin is a venous dilator that is used in the perioperative environment to control hypertension and for patients with unstable angina or congestive heart failure associated with acute myocardial infarction

Antiarrhythmics

Antiarrhythmics restore normal cardiac rhythm and conduction.

Cardiac glycosides

Classification: Cardiac glycosides are antiarrhythmic.

Action: Cardiac glycosides increase the level of calcium inside the cell inhibiting the sodium–potassium pump; this contracts the myocardial muscle and leads to increased cardiac output and increased blood circulation. This in turn slows the heart rate due to the decreased rate of cellular repolarisation of the heart. Digoxin can be used intravenously to treat mild to moderate heart failure and also for patients with atrial fibrillation. (Gahart & Nazareno 2014, pp. 386–9) When administered intravenously digoxin must be delivered very slowly over a minimum of 5 minutes to prevent arrhythmias. The patient must also be cardiac monitored and emergency equipment must be readily available. If there is an increase in urine output and the heart rate is normal, then the drug is being effective.

Adverse effects: These include headache, weakness, seizures and digitalis toxicity. (Gahart & Nazareno 2014, pp. 386–9; Broyles et al. 2013, p. 319)

Cardiac stimulants

Classification: Cardiac stimulants are antiarrhythmic.

Action: Epinephrine (adrenaline) is a natural hormone of the body and is secreted by the adrenal glands. It is responsible for the 'flight or fight' response within the body and is also used as a first-line drug when cardiopulmonary resuscitation (CPR), airway management and defibrillation have failed in patients with ventricular fibrillation, pulseless ventricular tachycardia, asystole or pulseless electrical activity. Adrenaline is a vasoconstrictor and a cardiac stimulant. It increases the contractibility of the myocardial muscle, increasing heart rate, and increasing myocardial and cerebral blood circulation during CPR. It is administered intravenously for cardiac resuscitation at a dose of 1:10 000 or 1 mg in 10 mL and may be repeated every 3–5 minutes as required.

Adverse effects: Include bradycardia, cerebrovascular haemorrhage, fibrillation, headache, hyper and hypotension, pulmonary oedema, pupillary dilation, renal failure, restlessness, tachycardia, weakness and death. (Gahart & Nazareno 2014, pp. 456–9)

Central nervous system agents

The CNS is the main control panel to the physiological function of the body. Some of the IV medications that interfere with the CNS and other body systems include opioid analgesics, sedatives, hypnotics, anxiolytics and anticonvulsants.

Opioid analgesics

Pain management is a large component within nursing and you must understand the types of pain, the physiological responses to pain and what may be prescribed to relieve pain for the patient. Opioid analgesics are common IV medications; these are derived from the opium poppy grown in China, India, Iran and Turkey. Morphine is a naturally derived opiate from the opium poppy; fentanyl is a synthetic opioid. Opioids are CNS depressants and are classified as a Schedule 8 medication, which means that they must be locked in a secure cabinet and a RN plus either another RN or an EN is to sign out the medication. Chapter 1 has more detail regarding each schedule. Ensure that you refer to the local policies, procedures and guidelines within your health facility governing the administration of IV medications, including the scheduled medications. IV opioid analgesics are commonly used in the preoperative and postoperative environment.

Morphine

Morphine not only relieves pain but it also produces a feeling of euphoria and changes a patient's mood. It relieves pain by binding to opioid receptors in the brain and therefore inhibits

the transmission of pain impulses. Morphine (see **Figure 4.8**) is used for moderate to severe pain and can be administered as an IV bolus, through a PCA (patient controlled analgesia) pump or by continuous infusion. An EN needs to monitor the circulatory and respiratory status of the patient.

FIGURE 4.8 Morphine can be administered intravenously

Hospira, Inc.

Fentanyl

Fentanyl is 100 times more potent than morphine and its main adverse effect is respiratory depression that can outlast its analgesic effect. The respiratory depression takes effect within 7–8 minutes of starting the IV administration. The circulatory and respiratory systems must be closely monitored. (Gahart & Nazareno 2014, pp. 522–4; Broyles et al. 2013, pp. 167–74; Alexander et al. 2010, p. 280)

Sedatives, hypnotics and anxiolytics

This group of CNS depressants cause drowsiness, induce sleep and relieve anxiety.

Barbiturates

Barbiturates produce varying degrees of action from mild sedation to deep anaesthesia. They interfere with the transmission of impulses across the synaptic junction within the cells of the brain stem.

Benzodiazepines

Benzodiazepines reduce anxiety, produce sedation, relax muscles and act as an anticonvulsant. They are considered safer than barbiturates and are less likely to interact with other drugs. An example of an IV benzodiazepine is diazepam.

Anticonvulsants

Anticonvulsants suppress the start and reduce the length of a seizure.

Phenytoin

Phenytoin is chemically related to barbiturates. It acts on the motor cortex within the brain to stabilise and depress seizure activity. (Gahart & Nazareno 2014, pp. 966–70; Broyles et al. 2013, pp. 215–16; Alexander et al. 2010, p 282)

Electrolyte and water–balancing agents

A large part of nursing care is the monitoring and management of fluid and electrolyte balance. In order to maintain homeostasis there are some IV medications that may be required to restore this equilibrium.

Replacing potassium

Potassium is one of the most common **electrolytes** that needs to be replaced due to depletion within the body.

Potassium chloride is required to treat hypokalaemia caused by loss of body fluids through vomiting, diarrhoea or diuretics. Potassium is essential for the regulation of nerve conduction and muscle contraction, particularly with cardiac function. Therefore potassium chloride must be given with caution, and must be diluted as directed. (Gahart & Nazareno 2014, pp. 989–92; Alexander et al. 2010, p. 290)

Diuretics

A diuretic is a substance that promotes the production of urine and aids in the elimination of sodium and water from the body. It may be used in the treatment of hypertension, oedema and congestive heart failure. Two IV diuretics that are commonly used are frusemide and mannitol.

Frusemide

Frusemide is a loop diuretic also known as Lasix. It is used for the treatment of congestive heart failure. It inhibits the reabsorption of water and electrolytes within the body at the site of the loop of Henle within the kidneys, thereby increasing urinary excretion. Adverse effects include hypernatraemia, hyperkalaemia and hypovolaemia. (Gahart & Nazareno 2014, p. 570–3; Alexander et al. 2010, p. 289)

Mannitol

Mannitol is an osmotic loop diuretic exerting a diuretic effect through osmosis, elevating the osmotic pressure within the renal tubules, stopping the reabsorption of electrolytes and water, and thereby leading to increased excretion of water and sodium. An adverse effect of mannitol is that it can increase blood volume and pressure and can potentially lead to hypertension, pulmonary oedema and acute heart failure. (Alexander et al. 2010, p. 289)

Gastrointestinal agents

Common causes of gastrointestinal tract disorders are nausea, vomiting and peptic ulcers. IV medications that alleviate the symptoms of nausea and vomiting are called 'antiemetics'. IV medications that protect the lining of the stomach, prevent the development and alleviate symptoms associated with peptic ulcers are called 'proton pump inhibitors'.

Antiemetics

Antiemetics are used to treat nausea associated with CNS disorders, certain medications, motion sickness and radiation therapy. The two most common antiemetics that are widely used within the healthcare environment are ondansetron and metoclopramide. There are many other antiemetics, which are used for nausea and vomiting caused by cytotoxic drug administration, opioids, general anaesthetic and postoperative effects.

TIP BOX

Never administer an IV medication unless you know what it is used for, and know its adverse effects and its compatibility with other drugs and fluids. If you are unsure, always check with a pharmaceutical reference guide (e.g. *MIMS* or *Australian Injectable Drugs Handbook*) or ask your local healthcare facility's pharmacist.

Ondansetron

Ondansetron hydrochloride (see **Figure 4.9**) is a 5-HT$_3$ receptor antagonist that blocks serotonin in the vagal nerve terminal and in the chemoreceptor trigger zone, stopping the complex vomiting reflex. It can be given as an IV injection or an intermittent infusion. (Gahart & Nazareno 2014, pp. 881–4; Alexander et al. 2010, p. 290)

FIGURE 4.9 Ondansetron can be administered as an IV injection or an intermittent infusion

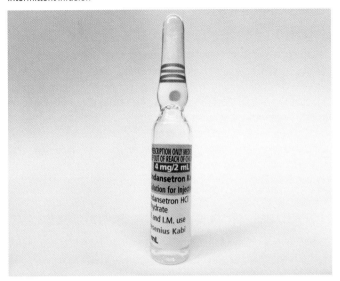

Metoclopramide

Metoclopramide hydrochloride (see **Figure 4.10**) is a dopamine antagonist that blocks serotonin and can be administered as an IV injection or an intermittent infusion. (Gahart & Nazareno 2014, pp. 792–5; Alexander et al. 2010, 2010, pp. 291)

FIGURE 4.10 Metoclopramide can be administered as an IV injection or an intermittent infusion.

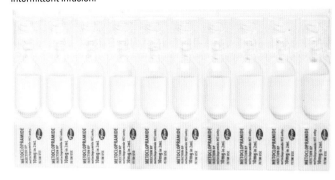

 Check each medication order carefully from the order written by the prescriber in the medication chart. Transcription of medication orders is dangerous and not considered legal.

CASE STUDY

Using generic names

Mrs Jones, a 75-year-old lady, has returned to the ward from the operating theatre following a total hip replacement. She states that she is feeling very nauseous and is holding an emesis bag. On the National Inpatient Medication Chart Mrs Jones has IV Maxolon and Zofran prescribed in the PRN section.

1 What are the generic names for Maxolon and Zofran?

2 What is the difference between the two?

3 What adverse effects do you need to be aware of before administering either Maxolon or Zofran?

 The potential problem of polypharmacy can affect IV medications. For more information relating to the problem of polypharmacy, see page 242 of *Foundations of Nursing*.

Proton pump inhibitors

Proton pump inhibitors block the final step of acid production, thereby supressing gastric acid secretion by the proton pump in the parietal cells.

Lansoprazole

Lansoprazole is used to treat duodenal and gastric ulcers, gastro-oesophageal reflux, hypersecretory conditions and upper gastrointestinal bleeding. Lansoprazole can be given as an intermittent or continuous infusion. Its adverse effects include headache, pain at the site of injection and nausea. (Gahart & Nazareno 2014, pp. 715–17; Alexander et al. 2010, p. 291)

Haematological agents

Anticoagulants are used to interfere with the coagulation pathway, inhibiting the clotting of blood and preventing further formation of venous thromboembolism (VTE), which is also known as deep vein thrombosis (DVT).

Heparin

Heparin is a commonly used **anticoagulant** that inhibits the clotting process by combining with other factors in the blood to inhibit the conversion of prothrombin to thrombin and fibrinogen to fibrin, thereby reducing the adhesiveness of platelets. A nursing consideration with heparin is that when administering a continuous infusion, coagulation tests (aPTT – activated partial thromboplastin time) should be performed every four hours. An adverse effect is bleeding and haemorrhage, therefore careful monitoring of aPTT levels is essential. (Gahart & Nazareno 2014, pp. 691–3; Alexander et al. 2010, p. 294)

Hormones and synthetic substances

Corticosteroids are synthetic substances that resemble cortisol, which is a hormone that the adrenal glands produce. They have metabolic and anti-inflammatory functions. Hydrocortisone is a corticosteroid that can be administered intravenously. Insulin is a hormone produced by the pancreas; however, for patients with diabetes mellitus, where the pancreas is not functioning or working effectively, a synthetic insulin is required to maintain endocrine function within the body.

Hydrocortisone

Hydrocortisone sodium succinate has metabolic and anti-inflammatory effects. Adverse effects of hydrocortisone include hyperglycaemia, Cushing syndrome, electrolyte and calcium imbalance and many others.

Insulin

Insulin assists with the transport of glucose and the use of glucose within the tissues. It also controls the storage and metabolism of carbohydrates, proteins and fat. Insulin can be used intravenously to treat and manage diabetes mellitus (Type I, Type II and gestational diabetes). (Gahart & Nazareno 2014, pp. 672–6; Alexander et al. 2010, p. 292)

Vitamins and minerals

Surgery, extensive burns, trauma or infection can alter vitamin uptake within the body. Also the current culture is consumed with high kilojoule foods that are high in sugars and fats but have minimal vitamins, minerals and fibre. Two examples of IV vitamins and minerals that are commonly administered are iron dextran and vitamin B1 (thiamine).

Iron dextran

Iron dextran is used for the treatment of iron deficiency anaemia. Iron is essential for the production of haemoglobin within the body. Haemoglobin carries oxygen from the lungs around the body, and carbon dioxide from the body to the lungs for it to be exhaled.

A nursing consideration regarding iron deficiency anaemia is the importance of monitoring blood loss due to gastrointestinal bleeding, trauma or menstruation. (Alexander et al. 2010, p. 294)

Vitamin B1

Vitamin B1, also known as thiamine, is essential for carbohydrate metabolism and other key reactions in the body. Thiamine requirement increases in direct proportion to the amount of carbohydrate being used for energy. It can be given as an IV bolus or added to most IV solutions and given as an infusion.

ACTIVITY

Piecing together the IV medication puzzle!
For each IV medication mentioned within this chapter, use information literacy skills discussed in Chapter 1 to search and write down alphabetically in a pocket-sized notebook the recommended dose, compatible fluids, administration (bolus, intermittent or continuous infusion) and nursing considerations. This notebook will be a good reference tool when you are working within the clinical environment. Ensure that you adhere your own scope of practice to the health facilities policies, procedures and guidelines regarding IV administration.

SUMMARY

Within this chapter the following concepts and issues related to IV medication have been covered:

- It is essential for an EN to understand the major IV medication agents, their pharmacological actions, adverse effects, monitoring and administration requirements to ensure the safety of patients requiring IV medication administration.
- Antibiotics are a common IV medication that is administered to kill bacteria. There are many different types of antibiotics.
- Patients who are being administered IV cardiovascular agents require cardiac monitoring and there must be appropriate emergency equipment available.
- Opioid analgesia help with pain management. Morphine and fentanyl are Schedule 8 medications, and require close observation of patient's circulatory and respiratory status. These drugs must also be locked in a secure cupboard and signed out by an RN and either another RN or an EN.

- Drugs that affect electrolyte and water balance include potassium and diuretics.
- Heparin is a common anticoagulant used to treat and prevent the risk of developing VTE.
- Corticosteroids and man-made insulin are synthetic replicas of hormones that are required to maintain homeostasis when glands that produce these hormones become ineffective.
- Vitamin uptake within the body can be compromised due to surgery, burns, trauma and infection.

REVIEW QUESTIONS

1. What is the difference between bactericidal and bacteriostatic antibiotics?
2. List one or two medications each for an antifungal, antiviral and antiprotozoal agent. Discuss how their action is different from antibiotics.
3. Beta blockers, vasodilators and calcium channel blockers are referred to as what type of cardiovascular agent?
4. Which type of IV medication can be administered, when prescribed, to decrease seizure activity?
5. What is the trade name for frusemide?
6. What is the function of a proton pump inhibitor?
7. What is an adverse effect of heparin?
8. Which hormone do corticosteroids resemble? Which gland releases this hormone? What is this hormone's function?
9. What is vitamin B1 also known as?

LEARNING OBJECTIVES

After completing this chapter, you will be able to:

- administer safely and effectively IV medication via bolus, infusion pumps, burettes, piggyback and syringe pumps
- understand what a bolus is and the relevant safety considerations to be aware of
- identify the different components of an IV line and its function
- explain how a burette works and the importance of its use from a safety perspective
- understand the different types of infusion pumps and their functions within the healthcare environment
- explain the primary use of the IV piggyback/tandem
- provide monitoring, care and maintenance to the IV cannula site and to the IV infusion line
- identify complications associated with IV cannula management and implement strategies to minimise these.

Introduction

IV medications are delivered on a daily basis by both RNs and ENs. ENs can prepare and administer IV medications as long as they have completed the appropriate elective unit of study and been deemed competent to do so. (Department of Education and Training 2014) It is the responsibility of the EN to practise within their scope of practice and become aware and comply with governing policies and the guidelines of their employer.

This chapter will give you the foundational knowledge and skill on the importance of care and maintenance of IV cannula management and the various ways to deliver IV medications and the delivery systems that you will come across as an EN.

Bolus

A bolus, also known as an IV push, is where a small volume of IV medicine or fluid is administered directly into the IV access port or into an already existing IV line. Many medications, including many antibiotics, can be administered via this method. The most common bolus is the 10 mL flush of 0.9% normal saline. The medication must be drawn up and administered over the correct rate in accordance with the *Australian Injectable Drugs Handbook* (2014) to prevent medication administration errors and complications (such as **speed shock**).

 For extra clinical information and practices related to boluses, see Section 7.6 of *Essential Clinical Skills* 3rd edn (page 230).

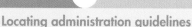

ACTIVITY

Locating administration guidelines

Locate an *Australian Injectable Drugs Handbook* and find three antibiotics that can be used intravenously. Write down the preparation, the IV bolus administration rate and the compatible fluids and drugs.

IV line

An IV line, also known as a giving set or administration set, allows for the administration of bags or bottles of IV medications or fluids directly to the patient continuously or intermittently, by gravity or through an electronic infusion pump. **Figure 5.1** (see page 59) shows an IV line with a spike adaptor to access the bag or bottle, a drip chamber, an injection port and a roller clamp to control the flow or rate of administration. The end of the IV line has a Luer lock, which is a locking system that secures onto the peripheral IV cannula (PIVC) or an attached needleless system bung.

For the IV therapies that are gravity fed it is important to understand the drip chamber. Drip chambers come in two different systems:

- macrodrip, which has a drop factor of 20 drops per mL and is the drip chamber most often used
- microdrip, which has a drop factor of 60 drops per mL and is used particularly for children where IV medication or fluid administration needs to be closely monitored.

Any IV medication can be gravity fed in accordance with correct administration rates; however, it is considered safer within many healthcare settings to use compatible IV lines with electronic infusion pumps to minimise the risk of infusions running too fast and so decrease the risk of air embolus. (Refer to Chapter 6 for infusion calculations on drip rates.)

EXAMPLE

Using a gravity feed line

Whether to use a gravity feed line depends upon the medication or solution to be infused, the acuity of the patient and the age of the patient. Always use the appropriate formula to calculate drops per minute, identify the drop factor of the IV infusion line and adjust the flow using the roller clamp until you have the desired rate. You must count the drops/minute for a full minute.

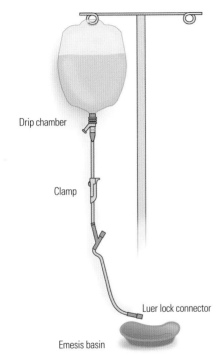

Drip chamber

Clamp

Luer lock connector

Emesis basin

Broyles et.al. (2013, p. 75)

Burette

A burette is a volume-controlled administration set that is connected between the bag or bottle of IV medicine or fluid and the IV line. It has a port at the top of the chamber to allow for intermittent medications to be mixed with a diluent prior to administration The burette allows administration of 1 to 2 hours of fluid volume. The burette can also be used for intermittent medication administration as it has a port at the top of the chamber, which allows the infusion fluid to be the diluent for the medication. You must ensure that medication and fluid compatibility is checked in the *Australian Injectable Drugs Handbook* prior to administration. **Figure 5.2** shows the various components of a burette.

ECS For extra clinical information and practices related to burettes, see Section 7.5 of *Essential Clinical Skills* 3rd edn (page 226).

FIGURE 5.2 Components of a burette

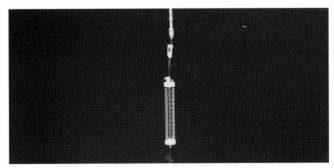

Broyles et.al. (2013, p. 75)

Infusion pumps

There are many types of infusion pumps, which are used for different infusions. They each use slightly different equipment, depending on the manufacturer's instructions. The three most common pumps used are the volumetric pump, the syringe pump and the patient controlled analgesia (PCA) pump.

The volumetric pump

The volumetric pump electronically controls and regulates the rate of administration of IV medications, fluids, blood and blood products, and nutrients intravenously or intra-arterially (into the circulatory system), subcutaneously or via the epidural space (see **Figure 5.3**). They can be used for both adults and children. Volumetric pumps should not be used for enteral feeding (via nasogastric or percutaneous endoscopic gastrostomy [PEG] feeding tubes) as there are other specialised pumps for this. Some volumetric pumps have medication libraries built into them in order to ensure safe medication administration.

> **TIP BOX**
>
> ### Check the type and brand of the volumetric pump
> Ensure you check with your healthcare facility to find out more information about the type and brand of volumetric pump that is used and the compatible IV infusion line that connects with the pump for administration.

FIGURE 5.3 The volumetric pump

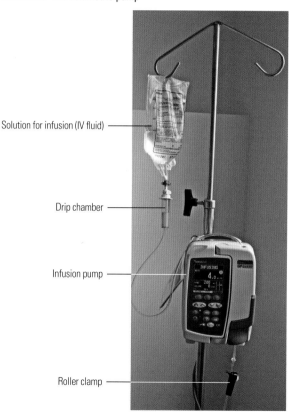

Solution for infusion (IV fluid)

Drip chamber

Infusion pump

Roller clamp

Brotto and Rafferty (2016, p. 126)

The syringe pump

The syringe pump, or syringe driver, is different from a volumetric pump as it holds a compatible, single-use Luer lock syringe that is depressed at a controlled and regulated rate to administer IV medicines, blood or blood products and nutrients electronically. Sizes can range from 5 mL to 50 mL (see **Figure 5.4**). You must check with your healthcare facility to find out more information about the type and brand of syringe pump or syringe driver that is used and the compatible syringe and Luer lock infusion line that connects to the syringe for administration.

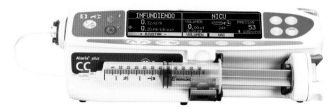

> **TIP BOX**
>
> ## Distinguishing between a syringe pump and a syringe driver
>
> The syringe pump is mostly used within an acute care environment to administer IV medicines hourly, whereas a syringe driver is often used in a palliative care environment and delivers either IV or subcutaneous medicines over a 12-hour or 24-hour period. (Wright 2011, pp. 112–14)

 It is your legal duty of care to ask questions about the use of a pump or syringe driver if there is any doubt, regardless of the seniority or experience of the person working with you.

The patient controlled analgesia (PCA) pump

PCA pumps allow patients to control the delivery of analgesia through the use of a PCA button (see **Figure 5.5**). A bolus dose is prescribed by the medical officer and the RN sets that rate into the PCA pump. The patient must be educated on the use of the PCA and the various features. The education needed for a patient using a PCA pump is shown in the tip box. The PCA can be programmed to have a 'lockout' period, which is the minimum time that must pass between bolus doses, even if the patient presses the button. It can also be programmed to provide a background administration of analgesia, which can be used in conjunction with the PCA button.

FIGURE 5.5 The PCA pump

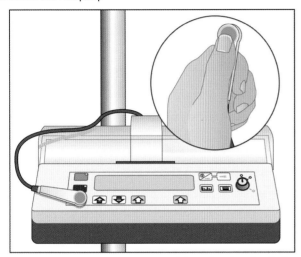

© Science Photo Library/Peter Gardiner

TIP BOX

Educating patients on PCA

Providing patient education on the use of the PCA is very important:

- Firstly, ensure that your patient is not unconscious or cognitively impaired and is not from a culturally and linguistically diverse community (CALD).

- If they are from a CALD community, ensure that you organise an interpreter to assist with the patient education. Always use an accredited interpreter who is familiar with medical terminology to ensure that the correct information is translated.
- Once you have established that your patient can understand instructions inform your patient about the reason why they are being connected to a PCA pump. For example, it could be for postoperative pain management.
- Inform them of the duration of the use of the PCA pump, which could be for 1 to 2 days postoperatively depending on how well the pain is being managed.
- Show them the PCA button, which they use to control the administration of their bolus dose, and inform them of the 'lockout' period, which is set to ensure there is a minimum time between two bolus doses.
- It is also important to inform your patient the frequency of observations that you will be performing to ensure safe administration of the PCA. Refer to your local healthcare policies and guidelines on observation requirements with PCAs.

IV piggyback/tandem

IV piggyback, or tandem, uses a primary and a secondary IV line (see **Figure 5.6**). The secondary line is used primarily for intermittent administrations, particularly of antibiotics. You must ensure that the IV medications and fluids that are being administered are compatible with one another. This can be confirmed by checking with the *Australian Injectable Drugs Handbook* or the health facility's pharmacist.

Care must be taken when disconnecting the secondary line, and always ensure good hand hygiene and asepsis. Refer to the section on the 5 Moments of Hand Hygiene and aseptic non-touch technique (ANTT) within this chapter.

FIGURE 5.6 An IV piggyback/tandem

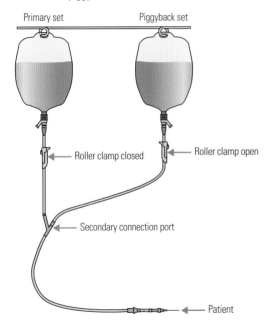

CASE STUDY

IV medications for treating sepsis

Mrs Andrews is an 86-year-old lady who has been admitted to the hospital from an aged care facility with sepsis secondary to a urinary tract infection and dehydration. Mrs Andrews is prescribed 1 litre of 0.9% normal saline IV at 125 mL/h. The doctor has also prescribed ciprofloxacin 400 mg 8 hourly.

1 What is the safest way of administering the IV fluids? What IV equipment will you be required to use?

2 What type of drug is ciprofloxacin, and what is it compatible with?

3 Using the *Australian Injectable Drugs Handbook*, describe how you will prepare and administer the ciprofloxacin?

4 List two possible complications that could occur with Mrs Andrews PIVC. Identify the cause, signs and symptoms and the nursing management of each complication.

Peripheral IV cannula (PIVC) monitoring, care and maintenance

An EN must be familiar with the monitoring, care and maintenance involved in providing safe and effective use of PIVC and infusion equipment. PIVCs are invasive devices that automatically put the patient at risk of healthcare-associated infections.

Infections can be acquired by **extraluminal** means, whereby 1–2 days after a chlorhexidine clean the patient's microflora and associated bacteria colonise under the dressing and migrate down the external side of the catheter from the insertion site to the tip of the catheter. This can be prevented by regular visual checks and monitoring of the insertion site and the dressing, ensuring that it is clean, dry and intact, and clear of any signs of infection.

Intraluminal acquired infections occur when the healthcare clinician has not adhered to hand hygiene, aseptic techniques and the healthcare facility's guidelines regarding monitoring, care and maintenance of the PIVC.

Monitoring

Part of monitoring the PIVC is ensuring that site inspection is a part of your daily care of the patient. Site inspection involves visibly checking the site at least once every 8 hours – checking the insertion site and surrounds for any signs of inflammation and infection, palpating the site for signs of swelling and obtaining subjective information from the patient (e.g. pain or discomfort). If a patient is on a continuous infusion, the site inspection needs to be every hour. When a patient is on intermittent IV medicine administration, the PIVC insertion site needs to be inspected before and after administration. To adequately inspect a site, an EN must be able to recognise signs and symptoms of infection and how to prevent and treat such an infection.

ACTIVITY

Terms related to PIVC complications

Define each of the following terms:

- Phlebitis
- Thrombophlebitis
- Erythema
- Pain
- Tenderness
- Swelling
- Inflammation
- Exudate
- Fever

Complications associated with PIVC

As PIVCs are invasive, it puts the patient at risk of various complications. Complications include inflammation (e.g. phlebitis), infection, infiltration and extravasation.

Phlebitis

Phlebitis is a form of inflammation of the vein. It has four different types – infective, mechanical, chemical and post-infusion. Table 5.1 shows the causes of each type of phlebitis.

ENs should know how to manage any signs of inflammation or infection (see tip box on this page).

TABLE 5.1 Types of phlebitis and their causes

Type of phlebitis	Cause of phlebitis
Infective	The site has an infection. This may be due to the clinician who inserted the cannula not using proper aseptic technique.
Mechanical	The inflammation is caused by the movement of the cannula, or poor stabilisation of the cannula.
Chemical	This is due to a reaction to the cleansing solution (e.g. chlorhexidine).
Post-infusion	This occurs 24–48 hours after the infusion and is generally related to infection.

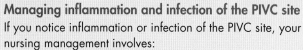

TIP BOX

Managing inflammation and infection of the PIVC site

If you notice inflammation or infection of the PIVC site, your nursing management involves:
- resting the affected limb
- elevating the limb if swelling is detected
- applying warmth (if no signs of infection)
- informing an RN and/or medical officer for further assessment and intervention.

Infiltration and extravasation

Infiltration and extravasation are also other common complications associated with PIVCs.

- *Infiltration* occurs as a result of a non-vesicant solution entering the tissues rather than the vein. This can be caused by the PIVC becoming dislodged from the vein due to patient movement or poor securement, or the PIVC having punctured the side wall of the vein. Infiltration when treated immediately does not have any long-term effects.
- *Extravasation* is infiltration with a vesicant solution. A vesicant solution has a pH of less than 4 or more than 9. Extravasation of a vesicant solution has long-term effects as it can cause burns to surrounding skin and tissue. Examples of vesicant solutions are chemotherapy (cytotoxic drugs), potassium chloride, radiologic contrasts and vancomycin.

TIP BOX

Complications associated with infiltration and extravasation of the PIVC

An EN should know the signs and symptoms and appropriate nursing management of any complications associated with infiltration and extravasation of the PIVC.

TABLE 5.2 Complications associated with infiltration and extravasation

Complication	Signs and symptoms	Nursing management steps
Infiltration	Swelling, pain and erythema	Stop infusion Elevate arm Notify RN and medical officer Document
Extravasation	Inflammation, pain, stinging or burning, erythema, swelling, irritation and blister formation at the infusion site	Stop infusion Notify RN and medical officer immediately Elevate arm Perform observations – blood pressure, pulse, temperature and capillary refill Document

Care

Prevention is the priority when it comes to PIVC management. In order to care for PIVCs the clinician must adhere to hand hygiene guidelines, aseptic technique and use of appropriate dressings; and also ensure patency of the PIVC and infusion lines.

The 5 Moments of Hand Hygiene

The World Health Organization developed 5 Moments of Hand Hygiene guidelines as illustrated in **Figure 5.7**, which Hand Hygiene Australia has embraced to decrease the risk of healthcare-associated infections. (World Health Organization 2009) Hand

FIGURE 5.7 World Health Organization: 5 Moments of Hand Hygiene

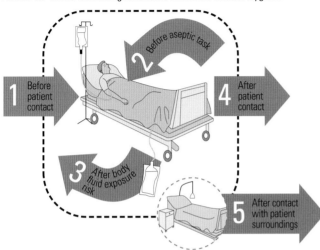

World Alliance for Patient Safety (October 2006, version 1), *Hand Hygiene: When and How*

hygiene should always be performed using soap, or antimicrobial solution and water or alcoholic hand rub. The 5 Moments of Hand Hygiene guidelines can be used in many different healthcare settings.

Aseptic non-touch technique (ANTT)

ANTT is a guideline from the National Health and Medical Research Council and provides a standardised process that is implemented within Australian hospitals and healthcare organisations to help reduce the rate of healthcare-associated infections. (National Health and Medical Research Council 2010) It is an approach to maintain asepsis during invasive clinical procedures and the maintenance of indwelling medical devices through the protection of **key parts** and **key sites**. ANTT should be used when performing dressing changes, and accessing or administering medications into PIVC.

Using ANTT when applying a PIVC dressing change

1 Perform hand hygiene with soap and water or alcohol hand rub.
2 Clean plastic tray with a detergent wipe or alcohol wipe. The plastic tray is the general aseptic field. Allow to dry. Gather equipment. Open necessary equipment (semi-permeable transparent dressing, 2% chlorhexidine with 70% alcohol swabs); keep the equipment in their micro-aseptic fields (their sterile packaging) and place them in the plastic tray. Ensure key parts are protected at all times.
3 Perform hand hygiene, put on apron and non-sterile gloves.
4 Remove old dressing and discard in contaminated waste. Remove and discard gloves.
5 Perform hand hygiene and put on new non-sterile gloves.
6 Handle non-key parts with confidence and protect key parts. Clean the insertion site in concentric circles with the 2% chlorhexidine with 70% alcohol swab, starting at the insertion site; clean to the edge of the dressing area. Allow to air dry.

7   Cover the insertion site with the sterile semi-permeable transparent dressing, allowing visibility of the insertion site. Secure extension tubing with sterile securing tap.
8   Remove gloves and apron and discard. Perform hand hygiene.
9   Document the reason for the dressing change, the type of dressing used and the date and time performed. Ensure to finish with your signature and designation as the clinician who performed the dressing change.

'Push–pause' technique

To maintain patency of the cannula and prevent mixing of incompatible medications and solutions a pulsatile flushing technique or push–pause technique with 0.9% sodium chloride is recommended. A pulsatile flushing technique increases turbulence within the lumen, which helps to prevent blood clots. Always refer to the health service guidelines regarding medical orders for 0.9% sodium chloride flushes, as it is a fluid that requires a prescription. When flushing always use a 10 mL syringe, as it produces a pressure of 10 psi. Infusion pressures should never exceed 25 psi as it can damage the blood vessel. Always flush prior to and after an infusion containing a different drug. Also flush every 24 hours if the PIVC is not in use; in this case you should discuss with the RN regarding the need for the PIVC to remain *in situ*. To prevent reflux of blood back into the lumen, always lock or clump the extension tubing while inserting the last 0.5 mL from the syringe; this is known as locking under positive pressure.

Maintenance

An important factor with PIVC maintenance is ensuring that there are no breaks in asepsis. Therefore, prior to accessing a PIVC, scrub the hub of the bung of the PIVC with a single-use 70% alcohol-impregnated swab and allow to air dry. All health services within Australia should be using a needleless-access port system; each health service's policy and guidelines and also manufacturer's instructions should be adhered to regarding these needleless systems.

A major patient safety issue has been identified by the Australian Commission on Safety and Quality in Health Care (2014) in relation to the administration of injectable medicines, fluids and the devices used to deliver them. If IV lines or syringes aren't identified clearly or correctly there is a risk of compromising the 5 rights of medication administration and putting the patient at risk. Therefore a national labelling standard has been developed to clearly identify what medicines and fluids are being administered. Each local healthcare service will have a policy regarding this. (Australian Commission on Safety and Quality in Health Care 2014)

Within this chapter the following concepts and issues related to IV medication have been covered:

- A bolus is a common form of administration method whereby a small volume of IV medication or fluid is carefully pushed directly into the PIVC via the IV access port.
- IV lines that are compatible with electronic infusion pumps are considered a safer option than gravity-fed lines because they decrease the risk of both air embolus and also the infusion being administered too quickly.
- Burettes can be used between the bag or bottle of IV medication or fluid and the IV line.
- The three types of pumps commonly used within the healthcare environment are volumetric pumps, syringe pumps and the PCAs.

- If a patient requires two or more IV medications to be administered, an IV piggyback/tandem approach can be used.
- It is a part of an EN's scope of practice to monitor, care and maintain the safe and effective use of PIVCs and infusion equipment.
- An EN needs to recognise signs and symptoms of a compromised PIVC and visually check the insertion site and palpate the surrounding skin at least every 8 hours, before and after every intermittent infusion and hourly for continuous infusions.
- It is essential that the principles of ANTT and the World Health Organization guidelines around hand hygiene are clearly understood and adopted.

REVIEW QUESTIONS

1 What is the difference between infiltration and extravasation?
2 Name the four different types of phlebitis.
3 What is the nursing management of inflammation and infection of a PIVC site?

4 What are the three most commonly used infusion pumps?
5 What principles should be adopted to prevent healthcare associated infections of the PIVC?

6 APPLYING FORMULAE FOR IV INFUSIONS AND DRUG CALCULATIONS

LEARNING OBJECTIVES

After completing this chapter, you will be able to:
- calculate volumes for safe administration of IV fluids and medications
- calculate and apply formulae for IV medications for adult patients
- calculate and apply formulae for IV medications for older patients
- calculate and apply formulae for IV medications for paediatric patients.

Introduction

This chapter contains the formulae that are most often used to calculate IV infusion rates and medications for administration. The chapter also describes the calculations used for the most common infusion devices. It provides details and examples for these calculations across the various age ranges. Both older and paediatric patients are at higher risk when receiving IV fluids and medications. Insulin infusion pumps are used in highly specialised situations. As these are mainly set up by medical specialists and specialised nurse practitioners, they will not be covered in this chapter. For all patients, calculations require very strict attention to detail and verification.

 For further information and practice relating to safety and calculations with IV medications, see Chapter 22 of *Foundations of Nursing* (pages 519–25).

 Additional supporting skills knowledge in this area can be found in Part 7 of *Essential Clinical Skills* 3rd edn (see pages 213–30).

Calculating volumes for safe administration of IV fluids and medications

The type of calculation used for safe administration of IV medications will depend on the method used to deliver the IV infusion. As discussed in Chapter 5, a number of different methods are available to deliver IV medications – bolus, infusion pumps, burettes, piggyback and syringe pumps. Essentially delivery is either by direct injection, gravity-fed drip infusion or volumetric pump machine.

TIP BOX

Knowing different methods of IV administration

IV injection (sometimes called bolus) and IV infusion are different:

- An *IV injection (or bolus)* is a direct insertion of fluid via a syringe, usually by the hand of the health professional.
- An *IV infusion* is a prescribed volume of a specific fluid going at a set rate over a stipulated time through an administration set controlled by gravity feed or a volumetric pump.

TIP BOX

Incompatibilities

No matter what medication or solution is being used, it is important to closely observe and note the fluid in solution – both IV fluid for infusion and the fluid used for medication reconstitution – for physical incompatibilities, as outlined in Chapter 2. The major sign is precipitation, where there is a change in the physical nature of the fluid and solid particles form.

For all calculations, you will need to know the volume of IV solution that the medication needs to be diluted into to be infused safely – this is often abbreviated as **VTBI** (volume to be infused). The amount of solution used to reconstitute the medication needs to be known as well. In total, these make up the full amount of IV fluid to be infused into the patient when giving a single dose of a prescribed medication.

Before starting to deliver medications, it is important to ensure safe delivery of any associated IV fluids. There is a high risk of error with IV fluids and medications, which demands careful observation and diligence when checking the medication and calculations. (Roughead, Semple & Rosenfeld 2013) This is a good time to check your 5 rights as outlined in the medication unit of competency, or whatever number of 'rights' that is required by your local policies. (Department of Education and Training 2014)

There are many different ways to calculate infusion rates, depending on the situation. The different types of systems of IV fluid administration are outlined in Chapter 5. This chapter describes some of the calculations used with these systems.

 It is your duty of care to be skilled in the calculation of all ways of delivering IV fluids. There are different supporting devices (or none) across different health service delivery locations.

 For extra information and practice related to calculations, see Chapter 22 of *Foundations of Nursing* (page 518).

Calculating for gravity-fed IV fluids in drops per minute

Figure 6.1 provides a basic calculation for most IV fluids that require the calculation of rate in drops per minute (**dpm**). This is common to all simple gravity-fed IVs that are regulated with a manual roller clamp. The most common drip chamber used in adults is the standard giving set which provides a **macrodrip** and delivers a drop factor of 20 drops per mL. There is also a

microdrip giving set which delivers a drop factor of 60 drops per mL; this is most commonly used in paediatrics and high acuity areas of hospitals. **Figure 6.2** shows the two different drip chambers.

FIGURE 6.1 Basic calculation for rate in drops per minute

1000 mL over 4 hours − convert to minutes:
    4 h × 60 min = 240 minutes

$$\text{Rate (dpm)} = \frac{\text{(mL)} \times \text{number of drops per mL (drop factor)}}{\text{time (minutes)}}$$

(over the numerator: total volume of fluid to be infused)

$$\text{Rate (dpm)} = \frac{1000 \text{ mL} \times 20 \text{ drops per mL (drop factor)}}{240 \text{ min}}$$

$$\text{Rate (dpm)} = \frac{20\,000}{240}$$

(in this example a macrodrip giving set is used, which delivers 20 drops per mL)

Rate (dpm) = 83.3333 drops per minute

Round this down to 83 drops per minute.

Where:

'number of drops per mL' refers to the use of either a standard giving set (macrodrip) which delivers 20 drops per mL or a microdrip giving set which delivers 60 drops per mL.

Brotto and Rafferty (2016, p. 134)

FIGURE 6.2 Drip chambers for delivering IV drops

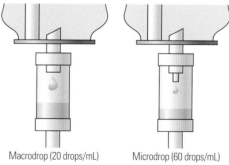

Macrodrop (20 drops/mL)   Microdrop (60 drops/mL)

Brotto and Rafferty (2016, p. 128)

Basic calculation for drops per minute

Shane Daniels is a 56-year-old man who will require IV antibiotics during his total knee replacement (TKR). The medical practitioner arrives to start his IV fluids and inserts an IV access line for the antibiotics. Fluids are ordered as shown on the fluid order chart (see **Figure 6.3** below).

There are two methods of calculating this rate – formula and ratio methods. (Brotto & Rafferty 2016) The formula method is the most commonly used and is used here. For further reading, the ratio method is detailed clearly in Brotto and Rafferty (2016) on page 134.

The task example is outlined here:

Using the formula for a standard macrodrip giving set of 20 drops per mL, the dpm that will deliver the fluids at the ordered rate via gravity feed can be calculated. The method for using this formula is as follows:

1000 mL over 8 hours – convert to minutes:

8 h × 60 min = 480 minutes

FIGURE 6.3 Shane Daniels's IV fluid order chart

Intravenous fluid treatment		Shane Daniels 20 Eric Street, Yapeen DOB 2/8/1959	Birthdate	

Date	Start time	Bot. no.	Volume	Type of fluid	Additives	Rate	Doctor's signature/ name	Signatures 1 Nurse 2 Checker
23/11/2015	Stat	1	1 litre	4% Dextrose in 1/5 normal saline solution	NIL	8 hourly	LSR Radford	

The next step is to insert this information into the following formula:

$$\text{Rate (dpm)} \quad \frac{\text{Volume to be infused (VTBI) in mL} \times \text{drop factor}}{\text{time (minutes)}}$$

$$\text{Rate (dpm)} = \frac{1000 \text{ mL} \times 20 \text{ dpm}}{480 \text{ mins}}$$

$$\text{Rate (dpm)} = \frac{20\,000}{480}$$

Rate (dpm) = 41.66

Rounding up = 42 drops per minute (dpm)

TIP BOX

When to round up or down

It is impossible to deliver a part of a drop. Round up if greater than or equal to 0.5. Round down if less than 0.5.

There are quick-reference tables available (see **Figure 6.4**) for looking up dpm rates for commonly used IVs with standard drip chambers. If you use these tables, be sure you still know how to calculate fluid delivery rates. This is an important safety mechanism for when there is non-standard equipment or when non-standard volumes or rates are prescribed.

 It is your legal duty of care to ask questions about a calculation if there is any doubt; regardless of the seniority or experience of the person that is doing the calculation with you.

FIGURE 6.4 Quick reference for drops per minute (dpm) rates

IV Rates *(for 1000 mL & 20 drops/mL)*

time	mL/hr	dpm	time	mL/hr	dpm
Q2H	500	167	Q10H	100	33
Q4H	250	83	Q12H	83	28
Q6H	167	56	Q16H	63	21
Q8H	125	42	Q24H	42	14

http://www.nursestuff.com.au/enurse-dosage-calculations-card

Calculating flow rate in millilitres per hour when time is known in hours

Sometimes it is essential to know how much fluid a patient is receiving each hour. Most volumetric pumps or syringe pumps require the input of two pieces of information – the VTBI and the flow rate (in mL per hour). **Figure 6.5** is the formula for calculating the rate in mL per hour, when the time for the infusion is known in hours.

FIGURE 6.5 Calculating rate in mL/h (when time is known in hours)

$$\text{Rate (mL/h)} = \frac{\text{total volume of fluid to be infused (mL)}}{\text{time (in hours)}}$$

EXAMPLE

Calculating mL/h with time in hours

Larry Browski is a 24-year-old man admitted to hospital requiring IV fluids for antibiotics. He is ordered the IV fluids shown in **Figure 6.6**.

FIGURE 6.6 Larry Browski's medical order chart

			Intravenous fluid treatment			Larry Browski 2/120 Farm Street, Coleyville DOB 12/6/1991		Birthdate	

Date	Start time	Bot. no.	Volume	Type of fluid	Additives	Rate	Doctor's signature/ name	Signatures 1 Nurse 2 Checker
12/10/2015	Stat	1	1 litre	normal saline solution	NIL	12 hourly	SG Gupta	

Using the formula shown in **Figure 6.5** (see page 75), the rate is calculated by inserting the information into the formula:

$$\text{Rate (mL/h)} = \frac{\text{Total volume to be infused (VTBI) in mL}}{\text{time (in hours)}}$$

$$\text{Rate (mL/h)} = \frac{1000 \text{ mL}}{12 \text{ hours}}$$

$$\text{Rate (mL/h)} = \frac{1000}{12}$$

Rate (mL/h) = 83.3 mL/h
(round down to 83 mL/h)

Calculating VTBI and rate (mL/h) when using an infusion pump

Sometimes you will need to calculate the VTBI as an hourly rate when infusion pumps are used.

Using the example of Shane Daniels shown in the example starting on page 73, the rate in mL/h required is as follows:

$$\text{Rate (in mL per hour)} = \frac{\text{VTBI in mL}}{\text{time in hours}}$$

$$\text{VTBI} = 1000 \text{ mL}$$

$$\text{Time} = 8 \text{ h}$$

$$\text{Therefore: Rate (mL / h)} = \frac{1000 \text{ mL}}{8 \text{ h}}$$

$$\text{Rate} = 125 \text{ mL per hour}$$

Calculating and applying formulae for IV medications for adults

Calculating and applying formulae for IV medications is different in each situation. This is why it is important to always have access to the latest edition of *Australian Injectable Drugs Handbook*. Shane Daniels's case continues here to illustrate the calculation of his IV medication. The example starting on page 77 shows a scenario for an adult.

The simple steps when giving IV medication to an adult are as follows:

- Check the medical order against the *Australian Injectable Drugs Handbook* to verify correct dose and check administration requirements and drug–fluid compatability.
- Gather and assemble required equipment.

- Mix the correct diluent and powder.
- Calculate the infusion rate for the additional infusion.
- Observe the patient, the fluid and the drip rate for any changes.

- Remove the additional IV line according to local policies and procedures.
- Document according to local policies and procedures.

IV medications for adults

Figure 6.7 illustrates Shane's medication chart where the medical practitioner has prescribed the IV antibiotics.

It is important to check the *Australian Injectable Drugs Handbook* when it is time to prepare the IV medication for

FIGURE 6.7 Shane Daniels's medication order

Intravenous fluid treatment	Shane Daniels 20 Eric Street, Yapeen DOB 2/8/1959		Birthdate	

Date	medication (print generic name)	Route	dose	frequency	indication	times	Doctor's signature/ name	Signatures 1 Nurse 2 Checker
23/11/2015	cephazolin	IV	1 g	6 hourly	infection	0600, 1200, 1800, 2400	*L Radford* *Radford*	

administration. The following information is from the online version of the handbook about **cephazolin**. The text has been bolded to assist you to develop your information literacy. In this case, the skill is to find the relevant parts within complex information.

The bolded areas are the ones relevant to Shane. This order is for 1 gram. The administration is most often an IV bolus injection, unless otherwise indicated.

PREPARATION

For IV use: **Reconstitute** the 500 mg and **1 g vials** and 2 g infusion bottle **with 10 mL of water for injections**. Or add 9.5 mL to 1 g vial to make a concentration of 100 mg/mL.
Powder volume: 500 mg – 0.2 mL, **1 g – 0.5 mL**

ADMINISTRATION

IM injection: Inject deep into a large muscle.
SUBCUT injection: Not recommended
IV injection: **Inject slowly over 3 to 5 minutes**.
IV infusion: Dilute the dose with 50–100 mL of a compatible fluid and infuse over 10 to 60 minutes. May be given as a continuous infusion.

The ampoule of cephazolin shown in **Figure 6.8** is available.

Undertake all medication administration checks (right patient, right time, right dose, right drug, right route and any additional 'rights' that might apply in your workplace).

The next step is to gather the required equipment.
- One ampoule of sterile water for injection (10 mL) (see **Figure 6.9**). It is important to *check that this is water* and not any other fluid.
- A 10 mL Luer lock syringe (see **Figure 6.10**)
- An alcohol swab (depending on local policy) (see **Figure 6.11**)

Latest evidence supports the use of a needleless system to draw up the water by using a blunt needle to draw up the fluid as the external surface of the water ampoule is not sterile. There are also proprietary needleless systems, as identified in Chapter 3.

From this point forward, the preparation of the IV medication is the same as the procedure outlined in Chapter 3 (page 36).

FIGURE 6.8 Ampoule of cephazolin

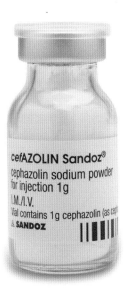

cefAZOLIN Sandoz®
cephazolin sodium powder
for injection 1g
I.M./I.V.
Vial contains 1g cephazolin (as ce
SANDOZ

FIGURE 6.9 Sterile water for injections

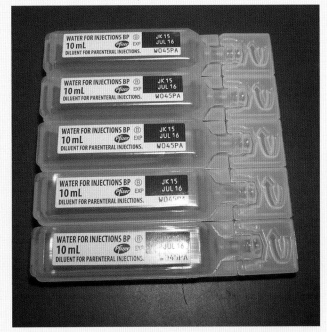

FIGURE 6.10 A 10 mL syringe

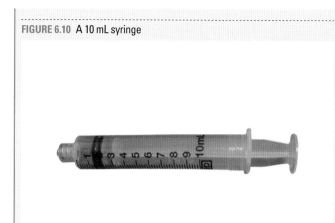

Source: Belynda Abbott

FIGURE 6.11 An alcohol swab

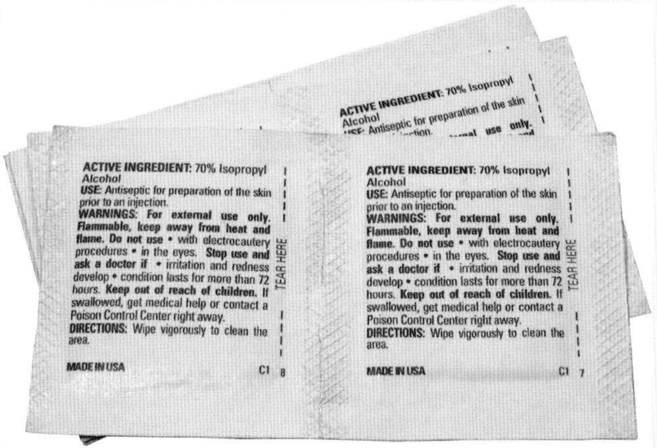

ACTIVE INGREDIENT: 70% Isopropyl
Alcohol
USE: Antiseptic for preparation of the skin
prior to an injection.
**WARNINGS: For external use only.
Flammable, keep away from heat and
flame. Do not use** • with electrocautery
procedures • in the eyes. **Stop use and
ask a doctor if** • irritation and redness
develop • condition lasts for more than 72
hours. **Keep out of reach of children.** If
swallowed, get medical help or contact a
Poison Control Center right away.
DIRECTIONS: Wipe vigorously to clean the
area.

MADE IN USA   C1 8

ACTIVE INGREDIENT: 70% Isopropyl
Alcohol
USE: Antiseptic for preparation of the skin
prior to an injection.
**WARNINGS: For external use only.
Flammable, keep away from heat and
flame. Do not use** • with electrocautery
procedures • in the eyes. **Stop use and
ask a doctor if** • irritation and redness
develop • condition lasts for more than 72
hours. **Keep out of reach of children.** If
swallowed, get medical help or contact a
Poison Control Center right away.
DIRECTIONS: Wipe vigorously to clean the
area.

MADE IN USA   C1 7

Jaimie Duplass/Shutterstock

Maintaining asepsis

As identified in previous chapters, it is *very* important to use ANTT (aseptic non-touch technique) when preparing IV medications. ANTT maintains asepsis of invasive clinical procedures and the maintenance of indwelling medical devises (such as an IV line) through the protection of key parts and key sites. (NHMRC 2014)

Calculating and applying formulae for IV medications for older patients

Older adults receiving medications are at increased risk of adverse effects and toxicity. The reasons for this include the older person's reduced capacity to clear medications from the body, a higher level of disease co-morbidities and medication complexity in this age group. (Roughead, Semple & Rosenfeld 2013)

The simple steps when giving IV medication to an older person are as follows:

- Check the medical order against the *Australian Injectable Drugs Handbook* to verify correct dose and check administration requirements.
- Gather and assemble required equipment.
- Mix the diluent and powder.
- Calculate the infusion rate for the additional infusion.
- Observe the patient, the fluid and the drip rate for any changes.
- Remove the additional IV line according to local policies and procedures.
- Document according to local policies and procedures.

The following scenario explores the detailed use of formulae and calculation for an older adult.

EXAMPLE

IV medications and the older adult

Elizabeth (Betty) Huxley, aged 87 years, has been in hospital for many days with a hip fracture that has been unable to be surgically repaired. She has developed fever and shortness of breath. A sputum sample was collected. The medical officer has diagnosed her with hospital-acquired pneumonia.

Before prescribing strong antibiotics for IV infusion in an older person, the medical officer will want to check their renal function to see if the person has enough capacity to clear the medication. Some older persons may require a lower dose if they have reduced renal function. There may also be a document in place (such as an advance health directive) to

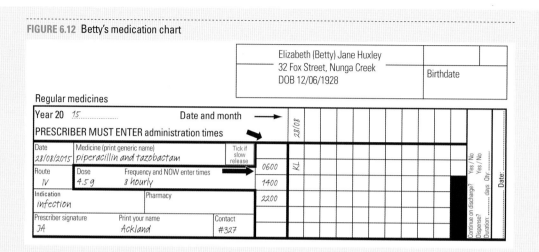

FIGURE 6.12 Betty's medication chart

support the older person's wish not to have IV antibiotics in a situation such as Betty's.

 Consider advance care directives for older persons.

Betty's medication order is as shown in **Figure 6.12**. You check the *Australian Injectable Drugs Handbook* with the RN (which is often local hospital policy for the first dose of any IV medication). The online version of the handbook provides the following information about

piperacillin and tazobactam. The text has been bolded for educational purposes.

PREPARATION

Reconstitute the 4.5 g vial with **20 mL of sodium chloride 0.9% or water for injections**. Or reconstitute the 4.5 g vial with 17 mL of sodium chloride 0.9% or water for injections to make a concentration of 200 mg/mL of piperacillin.
Powder volume: 4.5 g – 3 mL

ADMINISTRATION

IM injection: Not recommended

SUBCUT injection: Not recommended

IV injection: Not recommended

IV infusion: Dilute the dose with **50 mL of a compatible fluid**. Infuse over 20 to 30 minutes.

Australian Injectable Drugs Handbook 6th edn, SHPA (2014)
© The Society of Hospital Pharmacists of Australia

The next step is to assemble the required equipment and establish the correct reconstitution of the medication for IV infusion. The local policy is to use 0.9% sodium chloride for injections to mix this medication. You do this together with the RN, as you may be looking after Betty when future doses are needed.

The equipment will be the following:

- One ampoule of piperacillin and tazobactam (common trade name: Tazocin) 4.5 g (see **Figure 6.13**).
- One 20 mL syringe (see **Figure 6.14**) and a drawing-up needle (these come in blunt and sharp versions; the blunt ones are the safest to use to prevent needle stick injury) for mixing (see **Figure 6.15**)
- One 20 mL ampoule of normal saline (see **Figure 6.16**).
- One smaller bag of 0.9% sodium chloride, usually 50 or 100 mL. (Some facilities use 100 mL bags of normal saline; many others use burettes if IV fluids are already running.)

FIGURE 6.13 Tazocin (piperacillin 4 g and tazobactam 0.5 g)

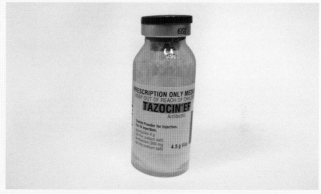

TIP BOX

ANTT

It is *essential* to use ANTT during the entire mixing procedure to prevent infection.

Mixing

1 Check you have the right drug and the right diluent by comparing with the medical order.

2 Wash your hands.

FIGURE 6.14 A 20 mL syringe

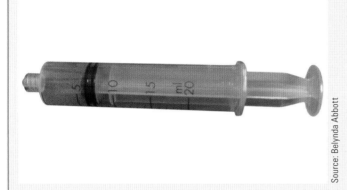

Source: Belynda Abbott

FIGURE 6.15 A drawing-up needle

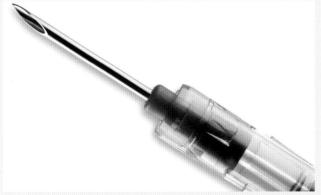

mholod/iStockphoto

FIGURE 6.16 Four 5 mL ampoules of normal saline

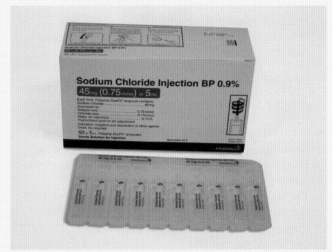

AstraZeneca Pty Ltd

3 Draw up the 20 mL of normal saline using a blunt needle and Luer lock syringe.

4 Apply the 18-gauge needle to the syringe.

5 Remove the lid of the vial of powder and cleanse according to local policies and procedures.

6 Pierce the rubber bung on the vial and begin injecting the normal saline while gently mixing until powder is fully dissolved in solution.

7 Draw full solution into syringe.

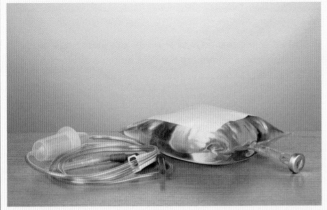

FIGURE 6.17 A smaller additional bag of a suitable IV fluid is often used for diluting IV medications

8   Insert IV tubing into a 50 mL bag and prime the line.

9   Following ANTT principles, wipe the injection port with an alcohol wipe, allow to air dry and then inject the solution into the 50 mL IV bag and gently mix until dissolved.

10   Attach the IV line to the appropriate connection on the primary IV line, or a burette could be used and the reconstituted medication injected into the burette.

11   Hang the 50 mL bag (with the 20 mL of normal saline – total volume now equals 70 mL) next to the original bag of IV fluid. Use the following formula to calculate drip rate to deliver at 70 mL over 30 minutes, or follow appropriate hospital policy.

$$\text{Rate (dpm)} = \frac{\text{VTBI in mL} \times \text{drop factor}}{\text{time (minutes)}}$$

Therefore, in this situation:

VTBI in mL $\times$ drop factor $= 70 \times 20 = 1400$

Time in minutes $= 30$

$$\text{Rate (dpm)} = \frac{1400}{30}$$

Rate (dpm) $= 46.66$

Rounding up, rate $= 47$ drops per minute (dpm)

12   Once the entire volume has gone through, remove the added IV line and discard.

13   Document on the medication chart as per local hospital policy.

TIP BOX

Continual assessment

It is essential to continuously observe the patient to assess their response to the medication. Report any itching, rash or other unusual symptoms immediately to the RN. This is particularly important with a first dose of IV antibiotics in any age group. It is also essential to monitor the fluid balance of anyone on an IV, and report any reduction in urine output.

Calculating and applying formulae for IV medications for paediatric patients

Paediatric situations require special attention to detail. There is little room for error in children's medications. This is particularly important with IV medications. Most large cities have specific children's hospitals with specially trained staff to care for children. Nonetheless, there are smaller urban, rural and regional hospitals that have a general paediatric unit for lower acuity cases. These situations may occur when there is a milder clinical concern, in which case it is better to keep the child near their home and family and treat the child in their local area.

The example below describes and follows a low-level paediatric case with IV medications.

EXAMPLE

IV medications and the child

Charlene (Charlie) is a 12-year-old girl whose mother (Katie) is a single parent living in supported accommodation. Charlie fell down the stairs when riding a skate board and sustained a large superficial laceration on her left leg last week. Katie cleaned and looked after Charlie's leg, but after a few days it became red, swollen and very painful. Charlie developed a temperature of 39.9 °C, so her mother took her to the GP who suggested admission to hospital with a diagnosis of possible cellulitis.

One day after her admission, you are to administer her midday dose of IV antibiotics. She has had two doses over the past 12 hours. Refer to Charlie's medication chart (see **Figure 6.18**). For this example, it is now 15 January 2016 at 11.30 am.

The first step is to check the *Australian Injectable Drugs Handbook*. The following excerpt is a quote from the handbook about **flucloxacillin sodium**. Text has been bolded for teaching purposes.

PREPARATION

For IM use: Reconstitute the 500 mg vial with 2 mL of water for injections and the 1 g vial with 2.5 mL of water for injection.

For IV use: Reconstitute the 500 mg vial with 10 mL of water for injections and the 1 g vial with 15–20 mL of water for injections. If the 1 g vial is too small to hold the 20 mL volume, carry out further dilutions in a syringe. Or reconstitute the 500 mg vial with 4.6 mL to make a concentration of 100 mg/mL or the **1 g vial with 4.3 mL to make a concentration of 200 mg/mL. Powder volume** : 500 mg – 0.4 mL, **1 g – 0.7 mL.**

ADMINISTRATION

IM injection: Inject slowly into a large muscle.

SUBCUT injection: Not recommended

IV injection: Inject slowly over 3 to 4 minutes.

IV infusion: **Dilute the dose in 100 mL of a compatible fluid and infuse over 30 to 60 minutes**.

IV use for infants and children: **Dilute to 50 mg/mL or weaker and** inject over 3 to 4 minutes or **infuse over 20 to 30 minutes. Infuse doses greater than 25 mg/kg to avoid phlebitis.**

Australian Injectable Drugs Handbook 6th edn, SHPA (2014)
© The Society of Hospital Pharmacists of Australia

You will note that the medical practitioner is required to write the dose calculation on the medical chart as illustrated in **Figure 6.19**.

This is best practice with the use of the Australian National Inpatient Medication Chart (NIMC – paediatric) that has been developed to improve safety. (Australian Commission on Safety and Quality in Health Care 2014)

It is an important learning tool and safety check in nursing to check the accuracy of this calculation. The following example from Charlie's medication order will illustrate the calculation (see **Figure 6.19**).

Current information at hand:
- Dose calculation – 50 mg/kg/dose
- Charlie's weight – 40 kg

Therefore each dose to be given will be calculated using the formula:

$$50 \text{ mg} \times 40 \text{ kg} = 2000 \text{ mg}$$

$$2000 \text{ mg} = 2 \text{ g}$$

From this calculation, each dose for Charlie will be 2 g.

Recommendations in the *Australian Injectable Drugs Handbook* to dilute the solution to 50 mg/mL or weaker

FIGURE 6.18 Charlene Blahovec's medication chart

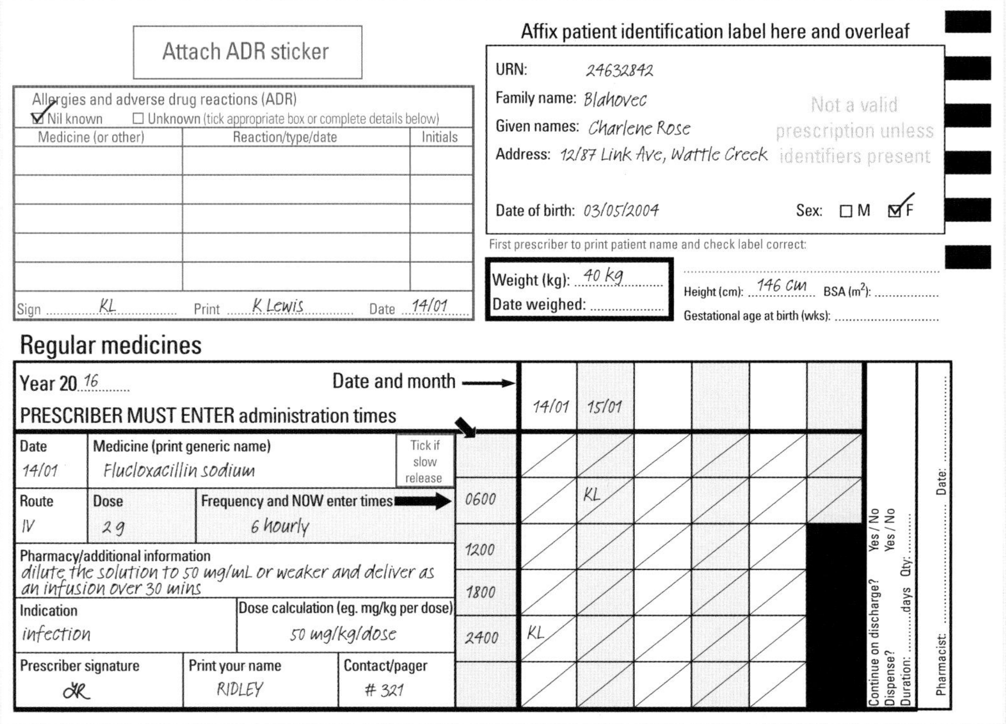

FIGURE 6.19 Information to be used to calculate Charlene's dose

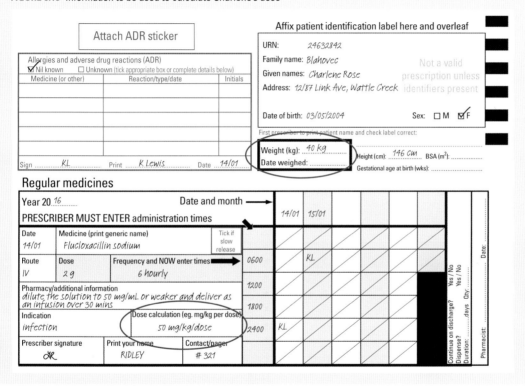

and deliver as an infusion over 30 minutes have guided local hospital policy to recommend the dilution of this IV antibiotic into a 50 mL bag 'piggyback' to get an even weaker dilution to protect vulnerable veins in children.

Your method and calculation will therefore be the same as the steps outlined for the scenario with Betty Huxley (see pages 81–6) with a different calculation.

TIP BOX

Check local policy

Each local policy will vary and it is important to check what the policy in your area states.

TIP BOX

Checking

Always check details at least *three* times before administering any IV medications – this means using the '5 rights' or the number of rights as your local policy.

In summary, the steps to use when giving IV medication to a child are the following:

- Check the medical order against the *Australian Injectable Drugs Handbook* to verify correct dose and check administration requirements

Once re-constituted, the calculation of the drip rate for this situation uses the same formula:

$$Rate\ (dpm) = \frac{VTBI\ in\ mL \times drop\ factor}{time\ (minutes)}$$

$VTBI\ in\ mL \times drop\ factor = 60\ (50\ mL\ bag + 10\ mL\ diluent) \times 20 = 1200$

$Time\ in\ minutes = 30$

Calculation is:

$$Rate\ (dpm) = \frac{1200}{30} = 40$$

Rate = 40 drops per minute (dpm)

- Verify dose with mg/kg/dose (or day) formula.
- Gather and assemble required equipment.
- Mix the diluent and powder.
- Calculate the infusion rate for the additional infusion.
- Observe the patient, the fluid and the drop rate for any changes.
- Remove the additional IV line and discard when finished.
- Document according to local policies and procedures.

FNE For extra information and practice related to calculations with children, see Chapter 22 of *Foundations of Nursing* (pages 518–19).

SUMMARY

Within this chapter the following concepts and issues related to IV medication have been covered:

- Detailed information about the application of a range of formulae for IV calculations has been explained, and illustrated by working through various applicable scenarios.
- General calculations as well as specific ones for adults, older persons and children have been shown.
- In every encounter with IV medications it is important to consult the latest *Australian Injectable Drugs Handbook*. Consider each situation unique. It is essential to check each

medication *three* times using the '5 rights' or the number required by local policies.

- Knowledge of local policies and procedures will support you in your practice.
- Never be afraid to ask questions – it is your professional duty to ask if you do not know about a certain piece of equipment or situation.
- Administering IV medications is complex; there are risks involved. Verification of information and close attention to detail is important.

REVIEW QUESTIONS

1 List six different methods for delivering IV medications.
2 What would you expect to report if you suspected an IV drug incompatibility?
3 Which fluids are counted when calculating the VTBI?
4 What is the difference between a microdrip and a macrodrip IV giving set?
5 Sarah Adkins is a 25-year-old woman who is admitted for dehydration. She has had an IV line commenced. She is ordered IV fluids as on the chart below in **Figure 6.20**.
   a Using the 'Basic calculations for rate in drops per minute formula' in **Figure 6.1** (see page 72) calculate the drip rate needed for Sarah Adkins.

   b Using the formula for calculating mL per hour in **Figure 6.5** (see page 75), calculate the rate at which IV medications should be delivered.
6 Luke Hindley is 42 years old and has been admitted to hospital following a serious hand injury at work. He is prescribed IV antibiotics as indicated on the medication chart below (**Figure 6.21**) for prophylaxis against infection. Calculate Luke's dose and administration using the *Australian Injectable Drug Handbook* information.

FIGURE 6.20 Sarah Adkins's fluid order chart

| | | | | Intravenous fluid treatment | Sarah Adkins 64 Newlands Road, West Waterland DOB 12.03.1990 | Birthdate | | |

Date	Start time	Bot. no.	Volume	Type of fluid	Additives	Rate	Doctor's signature/ name	Signatures 1 Nurse 2 Checker
02.02.2016	Stat	1	1 litre	0.9% normal saline	NIL	8 hourly	SK Kotecha	

FIGURE 6.21 Luke Hindley's medication chart

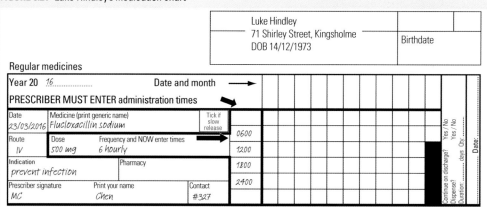

7. Alice McHale is a 90-year-old woman who has been admitted to hospital from home with a diagnosis of community-acquired pneumonia. Her IV has been inserted and she is ordered IV antibiotics as indicated on the medication chart below (**Figure 6.22**). Calculate Alice's dose and administration using the *Australian Injectable Drug Handbook* information.

8. Daniel Tillyard is a 10-year-old boy who is admitted to hospital for IV antibiotics for severe orbital cellulitis. He is 145 cm tall and weighs 50 kg. His IV is inserted and he is ordered IV antibiotics as on the medication chart in **Figure 6.23**. Calculate Daniel's dose and administration using the *Australian Injectable Drug Handbook* information.

FIGURE 6.22 Alice McHale's medication chart

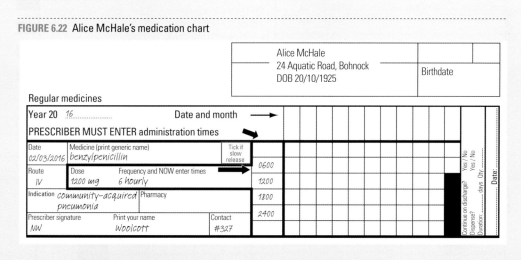

FIGURE 6.23 Daniel Tillyard's medication chart

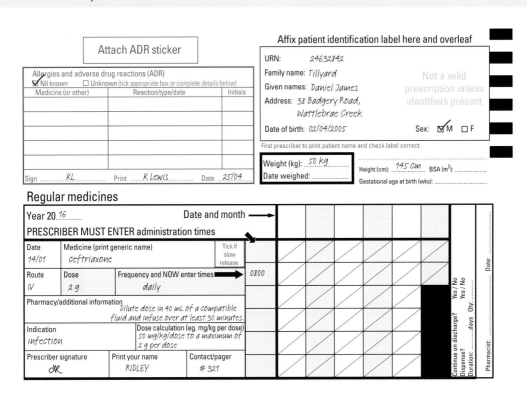

APPENDIX A: AUSTRALIAN AND NEW ZEALAND LEGISLATIVE REQUIREMENTS

Government laws ('Acts') cover the rules about medicines (and generally poisons as well) across Australia. Regulations are a set of mandatory requirements that are consistent with the Act and 'sit under' the Act for clarity of administration. The states and territories of Australia also have their own Acts and/or Regulations relating to medications. New Zealand has a national Act and national Regulation.

The following table lists the medication-related Acts and Regulations in Australia, across the various states and territories, and in New Zealand.

State	Act	State and Territory Regulations
Australian Capital Territory	*Medicines, Poisons and Therapeutic Goods Act 2008*	Medicines, Poisons and Therapeutic Goods Regulation 2008
New South Wales	*Poisons and Therapeutic Goods Act 1966*	Poisons and Therapeutic Goods Regulation 2008
Northern Territory	*Medicines, Poisons and Therapeutic Goods Act 2012*	Regulation contained under the Act
Queensland	*Health Act 1937*	Health (Drugs and Poisons) Regulation 1996
South Australia	*Controlled Substances Act 1984*	Controlled Substances (Controlled Drugs, Precursors and Plants) Regulations 2014
Tasmania	*Commonwealth Therapeutic Goods Act 1989*	Poisons Regulations 2008
Victoria	*Drugs, Poisons and Controlled Substances Act 1981*	Drugs, Poisons and Controlled Substances Regulations 2006
Western Australia	*Medicines and Poisons Act 2014*	Regulation contained under the Act
New Zealand	*Medicines Act 1981*	Medicines Regulations 1984

APPENDIX B: INTRAVENOUS CARE*

Venepuncture

Identify indications

Venepuncture provides access to the venous system via a needle for obtaining blood for diagnostic purposes or monitoring patient's response to treatment. Blood tests provide valuable information about a patient's nutritional, haematological, metabolic, immune and biochemical status. Medical staff order these blood tests. Accessing the venous system is an invasive procedure and requires a patient's consent. The patient's verbal consent plus their cooperation with a procedure is an implied consent. Written consent is not needed.

Most institutions consider venepuncture an advanced skill, and often have in-service and competency assessment programs for staff to gain the skills for establishing an intravenous access device or taking blood. Although the techniques are similar, intravenous initiation has more considerations and precautions of which to be aware.

Outline safety considerations

The venous system is a closed system which venepuncture breaches, providing an entry point for microorganisms. It is essential venepuncture is carried out using an aseptic non-touch technique (ANTT). Occupational health and safety principles should be followed to reduce needle stick injury or contact with the patient's blood. Various vacuum, non-touch and 'safety-needle' systems are available to assist in meeting these safety needs. Familiarise yourself with the safety devices available at your facility. Standard precautions must be maintained, and well-fitting non-sterile gloves should be worn. Determine the person's identity by asking their full name and date of birth and checking their identification band against the request form to ensure the specimen is obtained from the correct patient. Knowledge of the patient's medical history, current and recent medications and diagnosis is essential. If there is a bleeding disorder (e.g. pancytopenia or thrombocytopenia purpura) or a recent history of steroid or anticoagulant use, pressure needs to be applied to the puncture site for a longer time. Determine any patient preparation required (e.g. fasting) and check that it has been done. The medical staff must complete laboratory requisitions for all blood tests. The person collecting the specimen generally provides their name, signature and the time and date of collection.

Communicate effectively with the patient

Patient anxiety about the procedure may result in vasoconstriction. Giving a clear explanation of the procedure and working in a confident manner helps allay fears, anxiety and other potential complications such as haematoma. (Dougherty & Lister 2011) Many people have deep-seated fears of needles. Emphasising the

* Text extract from Tollefson, J., Watson, G., Jelly, E. and Tambree, K. 2016. *Essential Clinical Skills* 3rd edn, © Cengage Learning.

necessity and the benefits of the procedure helps people accept the unpleasant procedure. Do not be dishonest about the discomfort; give reassurance and emphasise it will be completed quickly.

Gather equipment

Gathering the following equipment prior to the procedure increases efficiency and patient confidence in the nurse.

- *The 'bluey'* protects bed linen.
- *Clean non-sterile gloves* uphold standard precautions and maintaining an aseptic non-touch technique.
- *A tourniquet* impedes venous return, engorging the veins and facilitating access.
- *An access device with an integrated safety system and a vacuum collection system (as per facility preference)* are used to draw the blood from the venous system. The access device is usually a 21 gauge needle, which enables the blood to be withdrawn without undue discomfort to the patient and prevents damage of the cellular components of the blood (RBC) from crushing (haemolysis). (Slade 2013) The Vacutainer system is specialised equipment used for accessing a vein. It consists of the plastic holder into which screws a double-sided needle and stoppered test tube with a vacuum.
- *Appropriate vacuumed test tubes* are needed. These attach to the vacuum collection system and automatically collect the required amount of blood. The stoppers on the test tubes are colour-coded for various types of diagnostic studies. Refer to the chart available on the unit for a list of the various tests and the appropriate test tube. Some contain preservatives, others

anticoagulants or coagulants, and some contain nothing. Collect the blood samples in this order: glass or non-additive tubes; coagulation; serum tubes with or without clot activator or gel separator; additive tubes such as gel separator; tubes which contain clot activator or heparin; heparin tubes; EDTA tubes. This minimises the risk of transferring additives from one tube to another. (Dougherty & Lister 2011)

- *A sharps container* receives needles following use.
- *Alcowipes* cleanse the skin prior to inserting the needle. Alcohol destroys microorganisms on the skin.
- *A gauze swab/low-lint swabs and bandaid or a pressure pad* are used to apply pressure to the puncture site.

Provide privacy for the patient by closing the bedside curtains or the door to the patient's room. Adjust the lighting to provide good illumination for the procedure. If the patient is in bed, raise or lower the bed to a comfortable working position to reduce strain on back muscles and improve access to the venepuncture site.

Assess the arm and site

Visually inspect the veins on both arms. Veins adjacent to an infection, bruising or phlebitis are not suitable because of the risk of causing more local tissue damage or systemic infection. Areas of previous venepuncture are avoided, reducing the build-up of scar tissue, which makes accessing the vein difficult and painful. (Dougherty & Lister 2011) When choosing the arm to be used for venous access be aware of such conditions as lymphoedema, a mastectomy or axillary node dissection on that side, an established intravenous access in that arm, an arteriovenous shunt or a haematoma at the potential site that precludes use of that arm for venous access.

The vein chosen for access is usually in the antecubital fossa – the median cubital vein is the common choice. Be aware that others may be more suitable, such as the basilic and cephalic veins. The median cubital, basilic and cephalic veins are straight and strong, and suitable for large-gauge venepuncture. The basilic and cephalic veins require stabilisation as they tend to roll. Ideally, preference is given to an unused vein, easily detected by inspection and palpation, patent and healthy. These veins feel soft and bouncy and refill when depressed. (Dougherty & Lister 2011)

To engorge veins, warm the peripheries and ask the patient to clench their fist. This increases blood volume in the venous system and makes access of these veins easier.

Perform hand hygiene

Performing hand hygiene removes transient microorganisms from the nurse's hands. This is an infection control measure preventing cross-contamination.

Gather equipment

Gather the equipment in a convenient position. Assemble the vacuum collection system. Position the chosen arm – extended to form a straight line from the shoulder to the wrist and well below the heart. A small pillow or towel covered with the 'bluey' under the upper arm stabilises it. The patient may be sitting or lying. Some patients feel very faint when blood is being taken and require the lying position to accommodate that.

Apply the tourniquet

Apply the tourniquet about 15 cm above the intended puncture site. Lay the tourniquet flat against the skin, clip ends together and tighten. Check the distal pulse to make sure you have not occluded an artery. If you are unable to locate a pulse, release the tourniquet and reapply. Leave the tourniquet in place for two minutes only, as prolonged tourniquet application may cause stasis, localised acidaemia and haemoconcentration. (Perry & Potter 2006) If you are unable to find and access the vein in two minutes release the tourniquet, wait a few minutes and reapply it.

Locate the vein

Locate the vein visually and, using the index and middle fingers of your non-dominant hand, palpate to determine the location and condition of the vein, distinguish veins from arteries and tendons and detect deeper veins. Palpating with the non-dominant hand increases the sensitivity and accuracy of locating the vein and also allows repalpation if the vein is missed to realign the needle (Dougherty & Lister 2011).

Ask the patient to open and close their fist slowly to increase the dilation of the vein. Pumping or doing this too quickly may affect the blood test results. (Dougherty & Lister 2011) Stroke the arm towards the tourniquet to dilate the vein. The vein should feel round and firm and spring back when compressed.

Don non-sterile gloves

Put on well-fitting non-sterile gloves as part of standard precautions.

Cleanse the area with an alcowipe

Cleanse the area with the alcowipe and allow drying. Using circular strokes outward from the intended puncture point avoids bringing microorganisms into the cleaner area. (Joanna Briggs Institute 2013a) Drying prevents stinging and discomfort when inserting the needle.

Access the vein and draw blood

With the access device in your dominant hand, stabilise the vein by stretching the skin taut above the intended puncture point using your non-dominant hand. The needle should be parallel to the vein and above it. The angle of insertion is about 15 to 30 degrees elevation to avoid going through the other side of the vein. The angle is dependent on the size or depth of the vein. Keeping the bevel of the needle upward also assists to avoid going through the opposite wall of the vein. Advance the needle through the skin and subcutaneous tissue and, gently but firmly, through the vein wall. You will feel the difference in pressure as the needle advances from the tissue through the vein wall (most commonly felt in adults, less often in children or in the frail elderly). A flash of blood appears in the hub of the needle or out of the tubing of the butterfly needle but not all Vacutainer needle devices. Reduce the angle of descent when this flashback is seen or when puncture of the veinwall is felt. Advancing the needle slightly into the vein stabilises the needle within the vein and prevents dislodgement during withdrawal of blood. (Dougherty & Lister 2011) If there is no flashback, withdraw the needle slightly as it may be in contact with a valve. If the attempt was unsuccessful, release the tourniquet, wait a few minutes and try again. Most facilities have a policy of only allowing three unsuccessful attempts, to protect the patient.

Firmly hold the access device in place with the non-dominant hand and push a test tube onto the back part of the access device needle using your dominant hand. The needle must be firmly anchored by the non-dominant hand to avoid dislodging the needle. The vacuum in the test tube will pull the required amount of blood into it. If no blood appears in the container (i.e. the vein was missed), do not use that container again as the vacuum will have been broken.

Release the tourniquet

Release the tourniquet to increase comfort and restore circulation. In some cases it may be necessary to release the tourniquet at the beginning of sampling to avoid inaccurate results caused by haemostasis (e.g. blood for calcium levels).

Withdraw the needle from the vein

Support the insertion site with gauze and withdraw the needle at the same angle it was inserted to avoid tearing the vein. Do not apply pressure to the puncture site until after the needle is fully removed to decrease pain on removal and prevent damage to the intima of the vein. (Dougherty & Lister 2011) Activate the safety device on the needle and place in kidney dish or sharps container.

Pressure is applied with the gauze for two to five minutes to assist clotting and to prevent bleeding and ecchymosis. Place a bandaid (ask the patient if they have any allergies to bandaids or tape) or pressure pad over the insertion site to continue the pressure to minimise bleeding. If the patient has fragile skin, do not use a bandaid or tape; rather, apply pressure to the puncture site until bleeding has ceased. The patient is advised to minimise activity with the involved arm and to maintain pressure on the site for five minutes. Observe the site for haematoma formation.

If needed, gently rock the test tube six to ten times to prevent haemolysis of the blood cells and to thoroughly mix the blood with any additives.

Remove and discard the gloves.

Label the test tube with the patient's information. Place the tubes in a biohazard bag and send the test tube and the laboratory requisition to the lab.

Clean, replace or dispose of equipment

Needles are placed in the sharps container for safety. Other items will be disposed of in the normal rubbish or contaminated waste bin. For efficiency, and collegial relationships, restock the tray as necessary with any equipment used.

Document and report relevant information

Documentation of blood taken usually consists of a brief notation in the progress notes including time, date, type of tests and patient response, the nursing care plan or patient Observation and Response Chart. Document and report any abnormal test results to medical staff.

Intravenous therapy (IVT) – assisting with establishment

Identify indications

Indications for intravenous administration of fluids are: 1) to restore fluid and electrolyte balance; 2) to maintain fluid and electrolyte balance; 3) for nutritional purposes (parenteral nutrition); and 4) to administer medications. Intravenous infusions introduce sterile fluids into the patient's circulation when the use of enteral fluids is not possible, sufficient or appropriate. Examples are pre- or post operatively, during trauma recovery or for IV medication administration. The insertion of the peripheral IV catheter (PIVC) is the responsibility of the medical staff or of nurses who have undergone specialist education and maintained their competency in cannulation.

Assess the patient prior to IV establishment

Assessment prior to IV establishment consists of several things. The patient should be assessed for baseline vital signs, allergies (to medications, iodine, latex, adhesive), medical diagnosis (especially heart failure, renal failure or bleeding disorders), planned interventions and general condition. Possible IV sites should be assessed for suitability. Take into account the patient's dominant hand (leave it free if possible) and avoid areas of flexion (antecubital fossa, wrist) and injury (mastectomy side, affected side of a stroke patient, arteriovenous shunt) or inconvenience (e.g. if surgery is proposed for the left shoulder, avoid the left arm/hand for IV insertion). Areas of localised oedema, cellulitis, dermatitis or skin grafts are avoided. Assess the size and condition of the veins and how often access will be needed (elderly patients or those with chronic diseases often have fragile skin and delicate veins). Children should have their IV access sited away from joints. Small, flat veins can be distended by warming them with warm face washers and keeping the arm dependent for a few minutes. Usually, initial IV access is at the most peripheral suitable site to leave the more proximal sites for subsequent access. Determine how long the IV access device will be needed – if it is more than a week, many facilities are now using central lines rather than peripheral lines. If there are no problems, PIVCs can remain in place for 72 to 96 hours (CHRISP&TC 2013; Fong 2014) before they are re-sited. PIVCs should be removed when no longer required or if complications develop. Review facility and state health department policy on the re-siting of PIVCs.

Communicate effectively with the patient

Demonstrate effective communication by giving the patient a clear explanation of the procedure. Many patients will be apprehensive about receiving fluids via an IV. Determine if they have had a PIVC before and what that experience was like. Some facilities use local anaesthetic to minimise the pain during insertion and reduce the associated anxiety.

Assist the patient to a position of comfort

Warn the patient that they may experience some discomfort during insertion or vein irritation during infusion and offer assistance if this occurs (warm compresses, mild analgesia as ordered). Discuss adverse effects that are common with the IV therapy and ask the patient to alert the nurses to any changes that they note following insertion of the IV line or change of an IV bag. Assess all patient concerns or complaints.

Gather equipment

Gather equipment prior to starting the procedure. Organisation increases your own confidence and permits a rehearsal of the procedure. It also increases the patient's confidence in the nursing care and minimises the time needed to accomplish the procedure.

- *Area IV trolley* is generally used to transport equipment to and from the bedside. Trolleys are usually stocked with all required items.
- *The intravenous fluid order sheet* with the written order is used to identify the IV fluid and amount required per 24 hours. The fluid order sheet has the patient's name, ID number, date of birth and doctor on it and is used during identification of the patient to ensure that the correct fluid and amount are being given to the correct patient.
- *The prescribed fluid* (one bag) is obtained from stock. Check the bag for an intact outer bag, date of expiry, type and strength of fluid and remove the outer bag/packaging. The inner bag may be damp from condensation. Check the sterile contents

of the inner bag for colour and clarity of the fluid by holding it up against both a dark and a light background. Gently squeeze the bag to check for leaks. Determine if additives are required. Two nurses (one must be a Registered Nurse) are required to check the fluid against the fluid order and sign the order sheet.

- *Required IV cannula (catheter), infusion port/connector, extension tubing and giving set.* Cannulae come in a variety of gauges, lengths and types. The doctor will determine which one to use. Generally the chosen cannula is the smallest size that can deliver the volume of fluid needed. The cannula will also have a safety needle system to reduce workplace health and safety (WHS) hazards. IV giving sets depend on the fluid being infused (crystalloids, colloids, blood, blood products), the patient and infusion pump being used. Each pump will require a specific giving set. For infusions not using a pump, adults usually have a macrodrip giving set with a chamber providing 20 drops per mL. Frail elderly people, children and infants generally require a giving set with a microdrip (60 drops per mL) chamber to make the regulation of the fluid more precise.

- *Other items* such as extension tubing and three-way taps and IV line sticker may be required.

- *Chlorhexidine gluconate 1–2% or isopropyl alcohol solution* are used to cleanse and disinfect the skin of the patient prior to insertion of the cannula. (CHRISP&TC 2013)

- *Non-sterile gloves* are required for protection of the person inserting the IV cannula or connecting the IV cannula to the line from body fluids, as a part of standard precautions.

- *The tourniquet* is applied above the intended IV site to reduce the flow of venous blood back to the heart. This distends the venous vessels, making insertion of an IV cannula more easily accomplished.

- *Extra tape* may be required to stabilise the IV line. The IV dressing will include tape for taping the IV line to the patient's arm.

- *Transparent IV site dressing*s enable continuous observation of the IV insertion site.

- *An armboard* may be required to stabilise the wrist or elbow of the patient to maintain a regular flow of fluid if the IV is sited close to a joint that, when flexed, might restrict infusion rates. Armboards are not comfortable and the IV site should be chosen to avoid any areas of flexion if possible.

- *The IV stand* is an extendable support for the fluid bag. Most have wheels attached to assist the patient with mobilisation. Many beds are equipped with an integrated IV stand to reduce the clutter at the bedside. In this case, a wheeled stand will be required when the patient gets out of bed.

- *Infusion pump* if one is to be used. Children, infants and frail elderly persons generally require a pump.

- *The sharps container* is taken to the bedside so that the used inner cannula can be immediately disposed of, thus reducing the chance of needle stick injuries.

- *A watch* with a second hand is needed to time the infusion rate if an infusion pump is not used.

Perform hand hygiene

Perform hand hygiene as a vital infection-control measure. The fluid being prepared is going directly into a vein and care needs to be taken in the preparation to maintain an aseptic non-touch technique (ANTT). Avoid touching of critical parts. Non-sterile gloves are used to comply with standard precautions.

Use general concepts and the 'rights of medication administration'

Use the 'rights of medication administration' to check, prepare and administer the fluid to the patient. IV fluids are therapeutic prescriptions and are thus treated as medications.

Prepare the giving set and check the IV pump

Prepare the giving set by removing it from its packaging and moving the clamp to just below (about 5 cm) the drip chamber. Tighten the clamp to prevent fluid flow until you are ready to prime the line and adjust the flow. Remove the protective cap over the spike on the top end of the drip chamber. Take care to maintain the sterility of the spike.

Check the IV pump for currency of maintenance and any manufacturer's instructions for programming the pump. Ensure alarms are working, batteries are charged and connect the pump to the mains supply. (Joanna Briggs Institute 2013b)

Spike the fluid bag

Spike the fluid bag after exposing the port on the fluid bag by pulling off the protective sheath. Rest the fluid bag on a table, hang it on the IV pole or hold it firmly under your non-dominant arm to ensure that the port is straight and the spike does not go through the sides of the port. Hold the side of the port with fingers of your non-dominant hand. Take care not to touch the outer edges of the port with the spike while firmly pushing the spike all of its length into the port.

Prime and label the line

Follow the manufacturer's instructions for specific guidelines on priming lines for an IV pump. Prime the line with fluid by hanging the bag of fluid on the IV pole. For lines with a drip chamber, gently squeeze and release the drip chamber until it is half-full. Open the roller clamp and allow fluid to fill the IV line. You may need to remove the protective cap at the distal end of the IV line (some caps permit priming while still in place). Hold the distal end of the line over the kidney dish and higher than its dependent loops so that air is expelled and fluid is not spilled. When the line is full and there are no air bubbles, close the roller clamp, reapply the protective cap and hang the line on the IV pole until it is needed. Place the required IV line label on the IV tubing (Australian Commission on Safety and Quality in Health Care 2012), noting the date of insertion. Make sure the dependent loop of the line is clear of the floor and the end is easily reached. If there are air bubbles, gently tap the line at the point where the air bubbles are, keeping the line between the bubbles and the drip chamber straight. The bubbles will dislodge from the line and ascend into the drip chamber. Raise the IV pole to a height not more than 1 metre above the patient.

Assist the doctor or cannulating nurse to establish an IV access

Assist the doctor or cannulating nurse to establish an IV access by assembling and preparing the equipment (use an aseptic non-touch technique), supporting the patient, inserting the primed line into the cannula hub and applying the dressing after any blood has been cleaned from the site. Most facilities permit only two or three cannulation attempts before a more experienced practitioner is sought.

Apply the dressing

Stabilise the cannula with your non-dominant hand and apply the transparent dressing using an aseptic non-touch technique. Carefully remove the adherent backing from one edge of the dressing. Apply the dressing from that edge, smoothing it onto the skin as you remove the backing. It should cover the insertion site and most of the hub of the cannula but not the adapter, again leaving the junction clear of dressing material. Write the date and time of insertion on the dressing. No tape should be attached to the IV cannula. (CHRISP&TC 2013)

Insert the line into an existing cannula hub

Put on non-sterile gloves. Hold the IV cannula hub and gently insert an infusion port into the cannula hub. The IV line is then inserted into the infusion port/connector. Insert the IV line into the IV pump and release the roller clamp on the line to allow fluid flow. Turn on the pump to run at the required flow rate. For IV lines without a pump, gently release the roller clamp to allow fluid flow through to maintain patency of the cannula.

Establish the ordered flow using the infusion pump

Infusion pumps differ from one manufacturer to another. Familiarise yourself with the infusion pump in use at the facility and ensure that the giving set is the one required for use with the pump. Close any safety clamps on the IV line. Open the door on the face of the pump. Thread the IV tubing through the pump according the manufacturer's instructions, usually in the direction of flow. Close the door. Turn the power on. As per doctor's orders, set the pump to volume per hour as appropriate to the pump. Determine the flow rate by calculating an hourly rate. Open the clamp so it does not impede the flow of fluid. Press the start button on the infusion pump. Check the flow to ensure that the pump is working effectively.

Formula for calculating flow rate: divide the volume (in mL) to be infused by the number of hours over which the volume is to infuse.

$$\frac{\text{Volume (in mL)}}{\text{Time (in hours)}} = \text{mL per hour}$$

For example, one litre of fluid in an eight-hour period is calculated by dividing 1000 mL by 8 = 125 mL/hr.

Establish the ordered flow rate for other IV giving sets

Calculate the flow rate to a 'drops per minute' rate by using one of the following formulae:

$$\text{Macrodrop giving set} - \frac{\text{volume}}{\text{time}} \times \frac{20 \text{ drops per mL}}{60} = \text{drops per minute}$$

$$\text{Microdrop giving set} - \frac{\text{volume}}{\text{time}} \times \frac{60 \text{ drops per mL}}{60} = \text{drops per minute}$$

Time the flow by counting the drops as they fall into the drip chamber for a one-minute period. Adjust the rate of flow by tightening or loosening the roller clamp. Again, time the flow, until the rate is as ordered.

Clean, replace and dispose of equipment

Clean, replace and dispose of equipment appropriately. The person inserting the cannula is responsible for the correct disposal of sharps and using the needle safety device after inserting the cannula and removing the insertion needle. This is disposed of in the sharps container. The tourniquet is washed, dried and returned to storage for further use.

Document and report relevant information

The insertion of an IV cannula is noted in the patient progress notes and nursing care plan. The type and gauge of the cannula, site of insertion, IV fluid type and amount initiated and rate of flow are recorded. The type and volume of solution is also noted on the fluid balance chart. A record is kept on the IV orders chart of the amount infused and the time bags were changed. Verbally report the amount of fluid remaining to be infused and the rate it is infusing during clinical handover. Insertion site observations are noted in the nursing care plan each shift (see skill 7.3). As a courtesy to oncoming staff, ensure the medical staff have ordered enough fluids to last until the following day unless the patient needs to be reviewed.

Peripheral intravenous therapy (PIVT) management

Identify indications

Intravenous infusion into a peripheral vein is a common therapeutic intervention in an acute care setting. Because of this, management of the IV and site are often thought to be routine. However, insertion of an IV line involves an invasive, painful procedure and establishes a break in the integrity of the skin, leaving a portal for infection. To prevent the premature removal of an IV line, and the infection or irritation of an IV site, proper care and management of the established line is imperative. Intravenous therapy is initiated for the purpose of providing a portal for the administration of fluids, electrolytes and medication.

To manage an IV infusion, the nurse must be aware of the solution ordered, the rate of flow ordered and if there are further solution(s) to be used after the current one is absorbed. This will be recorded on the IV fluid order chart.

Communicate effectively with the patient

Effective communication with the patient who has an IV *in situ* includes discussing the comfort of the site with the patient, reassurance that the frequent checks done on the peripheral IV catheter (PIVC) are a normal occurrence and requesting the patient to disclose any pain or other abnormal sensation associated with the PIVC.

Gather equipment

Gather equipment to increase efficient use of time and increase the confidence of the patient in the nurse's ability.
- *IV risk assessment tool or phlebitis assessment scale.*
- *The intravenous fluid order sheet* (often left at the patient's bedside) will have the solution, rate and doctor's signature. A fluid balance chart is also required.
- *A watch* with a second hand is used to time the flow of IV fluids if an infusion pump is not used.

Perform hand hygiene

Perform hand hygiene to remove transient microorganisms and reduce cross-contamination. Hand hygiene remains the single most effective measure for the prevention of hospital-acquired infection.

Assess the patient with a peripheral IV catheter (PIVC)

Assessment of a patient with a PIVC should be a continuous assessment if they are receiving IV fluid and the insertion site should be checked at least once a shift and prior to any administration of IV medication. (CHRISP&TC 2013) Continuous assessment includes monitoring of the IV flow rate, plus assessment of the patient. CHRISP&TC (2013) recommends checking the IV site hourly if there is a continuous infusion.

- *IV site* – The IV insertion site is assessed using the facility risk assessment and/or phlebitis assessment tool. A rating score is given for the site according to pain, redness (erythema) and oedema. Further advanced symptoms of streak formation, palpable vein or discharge are also scored. The score will determine the ongoing response and management of the IV site. (Sayakkara 2014) Other observations of the site include assessment for infiltration, indicated by discomfort, blanching, coolness of skin and a slow IV rate. (Fong 2014) The results of this assessment should be recorded on the nursing care plan or other IV documentation. Check the date of the IVC insertion and if the catheter needs to be reinserted. PIVCs can remain in place for 72 to 96 hours (CHRISP&TC 2013; Fong 2014) before they are re-sited.

- *Systemic assessment* – This includes monitoring for signs of circulatory overload, fluid volume deficit, septicaemia, hypersensitivity and pulmonary or air embolism.
- *Fluid and equipment assessment* – The established IV is assessed hourly to determine that it is infusing as ordered; the solution is the prescribed one; the rate is determined and altered if it is not the correct rate; the amount absorbed is calculated; and the amount remaining to be infused is noted. Also check required labels for IV administration set and any IV medications are correct and intact. (Australian Commission on Safety and Quality in Health Care 2012) Change the administration set if a line change is indicated.

During clinical handover, the IV site and IV fluids being administered should be checked by both the current nurse and nurse for the next shift.

Monitor the flow rate

Monitor the flow rate and compare it to that prescribed. The flow rate is monitored hourly, or more frequently if the rate ordered is very fast (over 120 mL per hour). Volumetric pumps ensure that fluid infusion is precise in millilitres per hour. Each pump will be subtly different and you will need to familiarise yourself with the model used in the facility. For areas where a pump is not being used, a flow rate control device (burette) should be considered for elderly, paediatric and/or critically ill patients. Some clinical areas may record the amount infused hourly on the fluid balance chart.

Some IV sites and cannulae are positional, causing the IV pump to alarm or the flow rate to change for lines without an IV pump. Maintain the height of the infusion at 1 metre or slightly more above the IV insertion site. Inspect the IV tubing for kinks or large air bubbles and ensure that the patient is not lying on it (and thus reducing or stopping the flow). Look for dependent loops and place excess tubing on the bed. Assess connections for leaks and tighten any loose connections.

Change a gown for a patient with an IV

There are IV gowns available that are designed to be easily put on and removed. These have fasteners (buttons, ties, Velcro) along the upper side of each sleeve. However, many patients prefer to use their own clothing. To remove a soiled gown or pyjama top, provide privacy and have the clean gown prepared (unfolded and in the proper orientation). With the assistance of a Registered Nurse (or advanced skills Enrolled Nurse) put the IV pump on pause, close the safety clamp and open the pump door to temporarily remove the IV tubing. Assist the patient to remove their unaffected arm from the original gown. Move the gown carefully over the IV insertion site and off the hand (so it is lying on the bed with the IV line still running through it). Take the IV bag off the IV stand and, keeping it above the level of the insertion site, slide the gown off the line and bag. Discard the soiled gown. Thread the clean gown or top over the IV bag and line (bag first) from the armhole to the wrist of the sleeve. Rehang the fluid bag. Carefully slip the gown sleeve over the patient's hand and insertion site and then help them to put their unaffected arm through the other sleeve.

Adjust the gown for comfort. The IV line is then returned to the IV pump, the safety clamp released and the infusion recommenced.

Assist a patient with an IV to ambulate

This consists of providing a wheeled IV stand and being mindful of the IV insertion site and lines. Many patients prefer to use the IV stand to steady themselves as they walk. Take care to assist the person from their unaffected side, to help them manage the tubing and to keep the IV stand far enough in front or to the side to prevent the patient from tripping on the wheels.

Change solutions on an established IV

Changing solutions on an established IV is similar to the initial establishment of IV therapy except that the line is already fully primed. Intravenous fluids need to be checked by two nurses as per policy (one is an RN) who both sign the infusion order. Check the IV fluid orders and bring the selected solution to the bedside and check the patient's identification ('rights of medication administration'). When the bag is nearly empty, perform hand hygiene and pause the pump, or if using the clamp stop the flow of solution. Remove the old fluid bag from the IV stand. Remove the spike by firmly pulling it from the old bag, taking care not to contaminate it. After exposing the port on the fluid bag by pulling off the protective sheath, spike the new fluid bag. Ensure that the port is straight and the spike does not go through the sides of the port. Take care not to touch the outer edges of the port with the spike while firmly pushing all of its length into the port. Hang

the new bag. Check the flow rate and pump programming, clear administered volumes and then recommence the IV pump. If an IV pump is not used, ensure that the drip chamber is half full and loosen the clamp to re-establish the prescribed flow rate.

Discontinue IV therapy

Clean gloves are used for this procedure. You will also require a dry sterile gauze swab and a small sterile dressing and tape. Bring this to the bedside in a kidney dish. Wash your hands. Open the gauze swab and the dressing. Cut a 10 cm length of tape and secure it by one edge in a handy place. Turn off the pump and clamp the tubing so no fluid can flow out onto the patient/bed. Put on the gloves. Carefully remove the tape securing the line and cannula, while holding the cannula firmly in place to prevent damage to the vein and keeping the skin taut to reduce the pull on the patient's skin as the tape is removed. Remove the dressing and discard into the kidney dish. Use the gauze square to support the insertion site. Pull the cannula or needle out along the line of the vein to avoid injury to the vein. Apply firm pressure to the insertion site with the gauze square for two to three minutes (the patient may do this if willing). Check the end of the cannula to make sure it is intact. Dress the site using a small sterile pressure dressing and the prepared tape. Advise the patient to call the nurse if bleeding occurs. If this happens, apply pressure and a new dressing. The site should be rechecked 15 minutes post removal. Place the used dressing, cannula and lines into the kidney basin and carry them and the fluid bag to the utility room for disposal.

Clean, replace and dispose of equipment

Excess solution in the discontinued IV fluid bag is emptied down the sink and the emptied bag placed into the garbage bin. The cannula or needle is removed and placed into the sharps container (needle) or contaminated waste (plastic cannula) along with the gloves and dressing material. The kidney dish is washed and returned to storage.

Document and report relevant information

The documentation for IV interventions is completed on the fluid balance chart and nursing care plan. Some facilities may have specific IV documentation. IV fluid bag changes, volumes infused and discontinuation of IV fluid are recorded on the fluid balance chart. IV site assessment is recorded on the relevant phlebitis assessment scale or IV risk assessment tool and reported during clinical handover. All fluids administered are signed on the IV orders chart.

Note: These notes are summaries of the most important points in the assessments/procedures, and are *not exhaustive on the subject.* References of the materials used to compile the information have been supplied. The student is expected to have learned the material surrounding each skill as presented in the references. No single reference is complete on the subject.

CASE STUDY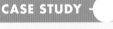

You are caring for Mrs Bowen, a 76-year-old lady who was admitted to your ward following emergency surgery for a fractured neck of femur. She is also dehydrated post operatively and has an IV line *in situ* for IV fluid. She also is receiving some IV medications.

1   Identify the specific nursing actions you would implement to manage and maintain her IV therapy.

2   Describe the assessment you will make of the IV site each shift.

3   What labels should be attached to the IV line?

4   The alarm sounds on Mrs Bowen's IV pump and she is complaining of some slight tingling and discomfort at the IV insertion site. When you check the site there is no redness, but the area is cool to touch, the skin appears blanched and there is some slight swelling.

   a   What is your assessment and response to these signs?

   b   Access an IV site risk assessment tool and chart these observations. What is the score?

APPENDIX C: REVIEW QUESTIONS

Part 1: General questions

General IV medication dose calculation

1 Mary Miller, age 58, is prescribed an 8 mg IV bolus injection of ondansetron. This is to prevent nausea associated with her chemotherapy. Ondansetron comes supplied in ampoules containing 4 mg in 2 mL. Calculate how many mL should be slowly administered in this IV bolus.

2 Holly McLennan, age 62, is prescribed IV ceftriaxone 2 g 8 hourly for a severe diverticular infection. The only stock available when you go to prepare the medication is vials of powder containing 500 mg of ceftriaxone. Calculate how many vials of this medication you will use to prepare the prescribed dose.

3 Kevin Jones, age 47, is prescribed IV flucloxacillin 2 g 6 hourly for a post operative infection after major surgery. The medication stock on hand holds 1 g per vial for mixing with diluent. Calculate the number of vials you will use to prepare the prescribed dose.

4 Timothy Gan, age 38, is prescribed 40 mg of omeprazole IV 8 hourly for a bleeding gastric ulcer. The medication stock on hand is in 20 mg vials. How many vials will you use?

5 You are working in operating theatre assisting the anaesthetist. Margaret Keating, age 79, is having a hip replacement. The medical order is to prepare for intra-operative administration of IV cephazolin 1.5 g as a single dose. You have on hand the following vials for mixing with diluent: 500 mg, 1 g and 2 g vials. Calculate which strength and how many vials you would use for this dose.

IV medication dose calculation using powders that need reconstitution

You are now preparing to give Holly McLennan's IV ceftriaxone 2 g from the vials containing 500 mg of ceftriaxone. The dosage and administration guide says to dilute 500 mg vial with 5 mL of water for injections. Answer the following questions:

6 How many millilitres of sterile water for injection will you use to dilute the 2 g dose in total?

7 What would be the final volume for administration after dilution?

Kevin Jones needs his 1800 hrs dose of IV flucloxacillin 2 g. The dosage and administration guide says to mix 1 g vial with 20 mL of water for injections. Answer the following questions:

8 How many mL of sterile water for injection will you use to dilute the 2 g dose in total?

9 What would be the final volume for administration after dilution?

10 In either of the above scenarios, does it matter if you dilute this further into a burette or larger amount of fluid? If, so why? If not, why not?

Part 2: IV infusion rate calculations

Using the following formulae, calculate the IV drip rate and infusion rate in mL per hour in the following situations. All calculations are using the standard 20 drops per mL giving set.

$$\text{Rate (dpm)} = \frac{\text{volume to be infused (VTBI) in mL} \times \text{drop factor}}{\text{time (minutes)}}$$

$$\text{Rate (in mL per hour)} = \frac{\text{VTBI in mL}}{\text{time in hours}}$$

You check the medical order and it is to give 2 g of ceftriaxone IV to Holly McLennan. You have diluted the 2 g into 20 mL of sterile water for injection as required by the dosage and administration information at hand. You note that Holly has a burette on her line. You ask the RN and she says that she has been having it further diluted to 50 mL in the burette over 30 minutes.

1 Calculate the drip rate for this 50 mL in drops per minute.

2 Calculate the drip rate for this 50 mL in mL per hour.

You check the medical order and it is to give 2 g of flucloxacillin IV to Kevin Jones. You have diluted the 2 g into 40 mL of water for injections as required by your information at hand. Kevin also has a burette on his line and you are asked to further dilute this amount into 100 mL over 30 minutes.

3 Calculate the drip rate for this 100 mL in drops per minute.

4 Calculate the drip rate for this 100 mL in mL per hour.

You are specialling a patient in the emergency department (ED) who is waiting for a bed. She is ordered 1 g of IV vancomycin to be infused in 500 mL over two hours. The RN does the calculation, as she is responsible for giving this medication according to hospital policy. She is mixing the drug in a 500 mL bag of fluid. She asks you to check the calculation with her.

5 What would be the hourly rate to infuse this amount over two hours?

6 What would be the drop rate to infuse this amount over two hours?

You dilute and prepare, according to the dosage and administration information, an ordered 500 mg dose of ampicillin sodium in a 100 mL bag of normal saline. This amount is to be infused over 30 minutes, as written by the medical practitioner.

7 Calculate the hourly rate to infuse this amount over 30 minutes.

8 Calculate the drop rate to infuse this amount over 30 minutes.

The medical order is checked and you are to prepare and give routine metaclopramide 20 mg diluted in 100 mL of normal saline over 30 minutes.

9 Identify the hourly rate to infuse this amount over 30 minutes.

10 Identify the drop rate to infuse this amount over 30 minutes.

Part 3: Case studies

Case 1

Amber Page is a 47-year-old retired teacher who is in the palliative care unit where you work as an EN. She is in the terminal stages of bowel cancer. She drifts in and out of consciousness and has a nasogastric tube on free drainage as she cannot take any more oral food and fluids. She has ice chips and mouth toilets. She is on IV fluids and receives her medications IV.

You have completed your unit for IV medications during your EN course and have undertaken the compulsory training and supervision to give IV medications under the direction of an RN within your organisation.

Her medication chart shows that she has been prescribed 8 mg ondansetron (Zofran) 8 hourly to prevent any nausea or vomiting.

You check the ampoule and it says: Ondansetron 4 mg/2 mL. You calculate the amount you would give using the simple dose calculation method:

$$\frac{\text{Strength required}}{\text{Strength in stock}} \times \frac{\text{Volume}}{1}$$

This is calculated as:

$$\frac{8}{4} \times 2 = 4$$

Therefore, you would give 4 mL for the 8 mg dose.

After looking up **ondansetron** in the *Australian Injectable Drugs Handbook*, you find the following information. Use this information to determine how you would give this IV medication.

ADMINISTRATION

IV injection: Inject doses of up to 8 mg over at least 30 seconds and preferably over 2 to 5 minutes.

STABILITY

Ampoule: Store below 30 °C. Protect from light.
Diluted solution: Stable for 24 hours at 2 to 8 °C.

COMPATIBILITY

Compatible fluids: Glucose 5%, glucose in sodium chloride solutions, Hartmann's, mannitol 10%, Ringer's, sodium chloride 0.9%
Compatible via Y-site: Compatibility information is available for ondansetron concentrations not commonly used. Consult the pharmacist, pharmacy department or medicines information service for more information.
Compatible in syringe: Compatibility information is available for ondansetron concentrations not commonly used. Consult the pharmacist, pharmacy department or medicines information service for more information.

INCOMPATIBILITY

Incompatible fluids: No information
Incompatible drugs: Aciclovir, aminophylline, ampicillin, azathioprine, cefepime, chloramphenicol, ertapenem, foscarnet, frusemide, ganciclovir, indomethacin, lorazepam, methylprednisolone sodium succinate, milrinone, phenobarbitone, sodium bicarbonate, sugammadex, thiopentone

Australian Injectable Drugs Handbook 6th edn, SHPA (2014)
© The Society of Hospital Pharmacists of Australia

1 What special precautions would you take with regard to incompatibility?
2 How long would you take to give this via direct bolus IV injection?
Circle one:
5 seconds   20 seconds   3 minutes   10 minutes
3 Is this a 'routine' administration of IV medication?

Case 2

Mason Bainton is a 68-year-old flight engineer who was admitted today to the medical ward where you work as an EN. He is admitted with the diagnosis of community-acquired pneumonia.

The medical practitioner commenced an IV line in the ED. During his time in ED, there was a medical order for 1000 mL of normal saline to be infused 8 hourly on a continuing basis. The RN on the night shift at admission gave his first dose of IV antibiotics (ceftriaxone sodium 1 g IV 12 hourly) and used a burette. Therefore, there is now a burette on his line. He is now due to have his second dose. It is now 1800 hrs on the 20 August 2015.

After looking up **ceftriaxone sodium** in the *Australian Injectable Drugs Handbook*, you find the information opposite. Use this information to determine how you would give this IV medication.

PREPARATION

For IV use: Reconstitute the 0.5 g vial with 5 mL of water for injections and the 1 g vial with 10 mL of water for injections. Reconstitute the 2 g vial with 40 mL of a compatible infusion fluid.

ADMINISTRATION

IV infusion: Dilute dose in about 40 mL of a compatible fluid and infuse over at least 30 minutes.[1] See SPECIAL NOTES

STABILITY

Vial: Store below 25 °C. Protect from light.
Reconstituted solution: Stable for 6 hours below 25 °C and 24 hours at 2 to 8 °C. The solution is yellow and may be slightly opalescent.
Diluted solution: Stable for 6 hours below 25 °C and 24 hours at 2 to 8 °C.

COMPATIBILITY

Compatible fluids: Glucose 5%, glucose 10%, glucose in sodium chloride solutions, mannitol 10%, sodium chloride 0.9%
Compatible via Y-site: Aciclovir, amifostine, anidulafungin, aztreonam, bivalirudin, cisatracurium, dexmedetomidine, foscarnet, granisetron, morphine sulfate, pethidine, remifentanil, tigecycline, zidovudine
Compatible in syringe: No information

INCOMPATIBILITY

Incompatible fluids: Solutions that contain calcium e.g. Hartmann's and Ringer's, parenteral nutrition. See SPECIAL NOTES

Incompatible drugs: Aminoglycosides – amikacin, gentamicin, tobramycin, aminophylline, azathioprine, azithromycin, calcium chloride, calcium folinate, calcium gluconate, caspofungin, chloramphenicol, chlorpromazine, clindamycin, dobutamine, dolasetron, filgrastim, fluconazole, ganciclovir, haloperidol lactate, hydralazine, imipenem-cilastatin, labetalol, linezolid, magnesium sulfate, mycophenolate mofetil, pentamidine, promethazine, protamine, sodium ascorbate

SPECIAL NOTES

Contraindication: Patients with severe hypersensitivity to penicillins, carbapenems and cephalosporin antibiotics.

Do not mix ceftriaxone with IV solutions that contain calcium because a precipitate can form. Deaths have been associated with precipitation of a ceftriaxone-calcium salt in the lungs and kidneys in neonates. Ceftriaxone is contraindicated in neonates receiving IV calcium-containing solutions. In other age groups, ceftriaxone must not be administered simultaneously with IV calcium-containing products but may be administered sequentially, provided the infusion lines are thoroughly flushed between infusions with a compatible fluid.

Do not inject intravenously ceftriaxone that has been reconstituted with lignocaine.

Each gram of ceftriaxone sodium contains 3.6 mmol of sodium.

1 Is the IV fluid ordered for Mason compatible with the ceftriaxone sodium ordered?
2 What fluids can be used to mix the powder before injection into the burette?
3 What size needle will you use to draw up the fluid to mix the powder?
4 How much fluid will you place into the burette to infuse the ceftriaxone sodium?
5 Identify what information you will place on an Identification Label that you will put on the burette.
6 Calculate the concentration of units per mL if you add the 40 mL prepared solution of ceftriaxone sodium and fill the burette to 100 mL.
7 Explain when you will the put the label on and take it off from the burette and why.

Part 4: Documentation

1 Identify a documentation error on the chart on this page with the date of the entry.
2 How should the date be written?
3 Identify a documentation concern with the time of entry.
4 How should the time be written?
5 Identify a documentation lack of clarity about the entry 'Feeling sick'.
6 How could you make this clearer?
7 Identify a concern about the entry 'since antibiotics'.
8 What would be more appropriate to describe 'since antibiotics'?
9 Using your answers and insights from the previous questions, what would you write after discussing this note with your RN?
10 Identify two unclear and inappropriate abbreviations used.

Allergies and Adverse Drug Reactions (ADR)		
Drug	Reaction Type	Initials
penicillin	anaphylaxis	QS
☑ Nil Known		

UR Number: 22019
Family Name: Spark
Given Name: Samantha Louise
Address: 39 Cofton Close, Hernani, NSW 2453
Date of Birth: 19 Feb 1999

Date and Time	Notes
Tuesday the 12th around 8pm	Feeling sick since antibiotics. Family asking questions. No answers given.
	Referred to doctor. Family concerned that IV is TKVO and the patient is RIB.
1015 hrs	

APPENDIX D: ANSWERS

Part 1: General questions

General IV medication dose calculation

1 4 mL
2 4 vials
3 2 vials
4 2 vials
5 One 1 g vial and one 500 mg vial; or three 500 mg vials.

IV medication dose calculation using powders that need reconstitution

6 20 mL
7 20 mL (could be slightly more, allowing for expansion with powder)
8 40 mL
9 40 mL (could be slightly more, allowing for expansion with powder)
10 It does not matter as long as you are using the full amount of diluting fluid and not less. You must also have accurate control over the period of time it takes to be infused.

Part 2: IV infusion rate calculations

1 34 dpm
2 100 mL/h
3 67 dpm
4 200 mL/h
5 250 mL/h
6 83 dpm
7 200 mL/h
8 67 dpm
9 200 mL/h
10 67 dpm

Part 3: Case studies

Case 1

1 Special precautions would be to check if the patient is now on any of the IV medications in the incompatible drugs listed. If they are, do not give medication and report to RN.
This includes the following:
Aciclovir, aminophylline, ampicillin, azathioprine, cefepime, chloramphenicol, ertapenem, foscarnet, frusemide, ganciclovir, indomethacin, lorazepam, methylprednisolone sodium succinate, milrinone, phenobarbitone, sodium bicarbonate, sugammadex, thiopentone
2 3 minutes
3 Yes

Case 2

1 Yes

2 Any of the following: Glucose 5%[1], glucose 10%[1], glucose in sodium chloride solutions[1], mannitol 10%[2], sodium chloride 0.9%[1]

3 18 gauge drawing up needle

4 40 mL

5 The answers are:

    a Patient name (given name and family name)

    b Patient identifier (ID), e.g. URN, MRN; Patient date of birth (DOB)

    c Active ingredient (medicine) added to burette

    d Amount of medicine added (including units)

    e Volume of fluid added to the burette (mL)

    f Concentration (units/mL)

    g Date and time prepared

    h Prepared by (signature)

6 2 g per 100 mL = 20 mg in 1 mL

7 Apply label immediately after injecting antibiotic into the burette. Take the label off as soon as the medication has all gone through. This is to ensure that the dose in the burette is fully given and that none is missed.

Part 4: Documentation

1 The full date should be provided.

2 12 June 2015 (any date that is clearly written like this)

3 Lack of clarity. Inappropriate use of time number.

4 2000 hrs

5 Vague symptom reporting. 'Feeling sick' does not clearly indicate what symptoms are being exhibited.

6 Reports 'feeling sick'. When asked, states she 'feels like she wants to vomit and is feeling hot'.

7 Vague time reporting. Does not give times or actual name of drug. Draws conclusions about the interaction between the time of the drug and the symptoms.

8 Reports 'feeling sick' since 1920 hrs. States that she thinks 'it is since the IV antibiotics'.

9 Reports 'feeling sick' since 1920 hrs. When asked, states she 'feels like she wants to vomit and is feeling hot'. States that she 'thinks it is the IV antibiotics'. Family asking questions and showing concern over history of allergic reactions. RN notified. Medical officer notified. BP, P, R and Temperature taken and recorded on observation chart. Jenny Jones EN

10 TKVO and RIB.

GLOSSARY

adverse drug reaction an unexpected or dangerous reaction to a medicine

agonist a chemical that binds to a receptor site and activates it to produce a biological response

air embolism bubbles of air that enter the venous or arterial circulation during a procedure that are large enough to cause an air-lock in the system and act as an embolism, causing tissue death

anaphylaxis a critical allergic reaction that is life-threatening; this should be treated as a medical emergency

antagonist a chemical that blocks a receptor site and stops it producing a specific response

antibiotics antimicrobial agents that are used to kill bacterial infections

anticoagulants a group of drugs that prevent clotting of the blood

aseptic non-touch technique (ANTT) an approach to maintain asepsis by protecting key parts and key sites from microorganisms transferred from healthcare workers and the environment

cellulitis an infection (usually bacterial) of the skin and surrounding tissues

diluent a fluid used to dilute medication in a solution

dpm commonly used abbreviation for 'drops per minute' when describing and calculating IV solutions

electrolytes ions within the blood and body fluid that carry an electric charge

enrolled nurse a nurse who has obtained a Diploma of Enrolled Nursing from a TAFE or a Registered Training Organisation

extraluminal outside the tube

gravity feed the simplest way of delivering short-term IV solutions. The rate is controlled by counting the number of drops. These are viewed in a chamber that is part of a giving set connected to a bag or bottle of IV solution

guideline a rule or piece of advice

information literacy skill in being able to differentiate and access good-quality information

intraluminal inside the tube

IV infusion a solution that is slowly injected via a gravity feed or other device into a vein

IV injection (or bolus) a solution that is injected via a syringe, usually by hand, into a vein

key parts critical parts of equipment that must remain sterile as they come in contact with key sites

key sites the area on the patient, such as an IV insertion site, that must be protected from microorganisms; these also include open wounds, including incisions and puncture sites

macrodrip a type of IV giving set that delivers 20 drops per mL of IV fluid. It is most commonly used in general adult situations

microdrip a type of IV giving set that delivers 60 drops per mL of IV fluid. It is most commonly used in paediatric and high acuity care situations

penicillins a group of antibiotics used to treat infections

peripheral line an IV line that has been inserted in the peripheral parts of the body, usually the arm, hand, leg or foot

pharmacodynamics the study of what a drug does to the body

pharmacokinetics the study of what the body does to the drug

phlebitis inflammation of a vein in the body

piggyback (or tandem) the use of a primary IV line with a secondary IV line used primarily for intermittent administrations, particularly of antibiotics

policies principles of action developed by an organisation, which must be adhered to

precipitation solids that develop out of substances that have been mixed in any liquid solution

priming the IV line an activity at the time of hanging an IV line where it is ensured that fluid fills the entire tubing with no air gaps

procedures series of actions developed by an organisation, which must be followed

receptor sites a site on the surface of or within a cell that is capable of recognising and combining with specific molecules

scope of practice actions and processes that nurses and midwives have been educated about, and are competent and authorised to perform

speed shock an adverse reaction to IV medications or drugs administered too quickly

toxicology the study of the negative effects of chemical, physical or biological agents on living organisms and the Earth

veins vessels in the body that return de-oxygenated blood to the heart

vesicant a drug that causes blisters and tissue necrosis when extravasated

VTBI (volume to be infused) a commonly used abbreviation to describe the full amount of an IV solution to be infused

REFERENCES

CHAPTER 1

Alexander, M., Corrigan, A., Gorski, L., Hankins, J. & Perucca, R. (eds) 2010, *Infusion nursing: an evidence-based approach*, Saunders Elservier, St. Louis Missouri.

Association of Colleges & Research Libraries of the American Library Association 2009, *Information literacy competency standards for higher education*, viewed 21 October 2014, http://www.ala.org/acrl/standards/informationliteracycompetency

Australian Nursing and Midwifery Council 2002, *National competency standards for the enrolled nurse*, viewed 16 December 2014, http://www.nursingmidwiferyboard.gov.au/Codes-Guidelines-Statements/Codes-Guidelines.aspx#competencystandards

Brown, S.A., Mullins, R.J. & Gold, M.S. 2006, MJA practice essentials – allergy 2 anaphylaxis: diagnosis and management, *Medical Journal of Australia*, vol. 185(5), pp. 283–9.

Department of Health Therapeutic Goods Administration 2011, http://www.tga.gov.au/

Koutoukidis, G., Stainton, K. & Hughson, J. 2013, *Tabbner's nursing care: theory and practice*, 6th edn, Elsevier, Chatswood NSW.

Merriam-Webster 2015, 'intravenous', *Merriam-Webster Medical Dictionary*, http://www.merriam-webster.com/medical/intravenous

Nosek, B.L. & Trendel-Leader, D. 2013, *IV therapy for dummies*, John Wiley & Sons, Inc., Hoboken NJ.

Nursing and Midwifery Board of Australia 2007, *A national framework for the development of decision-making tools for nursing and midwifery practice*, http://www.nursingmidwiferyboard.gov.au/Codes-Guidelines-Statements/Codes-Guidelines.aspx#dmf

Nursing and Midwifery Board of Australia 2014, *Explanatory notes: enrolled nurses and medicine administration Fact Sheet*, viewed 16 November 2014, http://www.nursingmidwiferyboard.gov.au/Codes-Guidelines-Statements/FAQ/Enrolled-nurses-and-medicine-administration.aspx

Queensland Consolidated Regulations 1996, Health (drugs and poisons) regulation 1996 Sect 58A, http://www5.austlii.edu.au/au/legis/qld/consol_reg/hapr1996340/

CHAPTER 2

Australian Commission on Safety and Quality in Health Care 2014a, *High 5s project: Assuring medication accuracy at transitions of care, Australian interim report, January 2010 – March 2013*, http://www.safetyandquality.gov.au/wp-content/uploads/2014/11/High-5s-Project-Assuring-Medication-Accuracy-at-transitions-of-Care-Aust-Int-Report.pdf

Australian Commission on Safety and Quality in Health Care 2014b, *Medication safety section*, viewed 25 June 2015, http://www.safetyandquality.gov.au/our-work/medication-safety/

Brown, S.G., Mullins, R.J. & Gold, M.S. 2006, 2 Anaphylaxis: diagnosis and management *Medical Journal of Australia*, vol. 185(5), pp. 283–9, viewed 1 November 2014, https://www.mja.com.au/journal/2006/185/5/2-anaphylaxis-diagnosis-and-management

Department of Education and Training 2014, *Training.gov.au. Unit of competency details*, viewed 11 December 2014, http://training.gov.au/Training/Details/HLTEN507C

Department of Health Therapeutic Goods Administration 2014, *Reporting adverse drug reactions*, viewed 11 December 2014, https://www.tga.gov.au/publication/reporting-adverse-drug-reactions

Frandsen, G. & Pennington, S.S. 2013, *Abram's clinical drug therapy: rationales for nursing practice*, Lippincott, Williams and Wilkins, Philadelphia.

Golan, D.E., Tashjian, A.H. & Armstrong, E.J. 2012, *Principles of pharmacology: the pathophysiologic basis of drug therapy*, Wolters Kluwer/Lippincott, Williams and Wilkins, Philadelphia.

Josephson, D.L. 2006, 'Risks, complications, and adverse reactions associated with intravenous infusion therapy', in D.L. Josephson, *Intravenous infusion therapy for medical assistants*. The American Association of Medical Assistants, Thomson Delmar Learning, Clifton Park, pp. 56–82.

Merck manual professional edition 2014, *Overview of pharmacodynamics*, Merck Sharp & Dohme, viewed 22 November 2014, http://www.merckmanuals.com/professional /clinical_pharmacology/pharmacodynamics /overview_of_pharmacodynamics.html

Merck manual professional edition 2014, *Overview of pharmacokinetics*, Merck Sharp & Dohme, viewed 22 November 2014, http://www.merckmanuals.com/professional /clinical_pharmacology/pharmacokinetics /overview_of_pharmacokinetics.html

National Institute of General Medical Sciences, Basic discoveries for better health. *Medicines by design*, viewed 22 November 2014, http://publications.nigms.nih.gov /medbydesign/index.html

Nemec, K., Kopelent-Frank, H. & Grief, R. 2008, Standardization of infusion solutions to reduce the risk of incompatibility. *American Journal of Health System Pharmacy*, vol. 65 (Sept), pp. 1648–54.

Royal College of Nursing 2010, *Standards for infusion therapy*, 3rd edn, Royal College of Nursing, London. http://www.bbraun.it /documents/RCN-Guidlines-for-IV-therapy.pdf

Smith, W. 2013, Adverse drug reactions: allergy? side-effect? intolerance? *Australian Family Physician*, vol. 42, No.1, January/February, pp. 12–16. http://www.racgp.org.au /afp/2013/januaryfebruary/adverse -drug-reactions/

Society of Hospital Pharmacists of Australia 2014, *Australian injectable drugs handbook* (2014), 6th edn, SHPA, Collingwood Victoria.

Society of Toxicology 2005, Special issue 2005, *How do you define toxicology?*, viewed 11 December 2014, http://www.toxicology.org /AI/PUB/si05/Si05_Define.asp

Westabrook, J.I., Rob, M.I., Woods, A. & Parry, D. 2011, Errors in the administration of intravenous medications in hospital and the role of correct procedures and nurse experience, *British Medical Journal Quality and Safety*, doi:10.1136/bmjqs-2011-000089

CHAPTER 3

Arcus, J., Gallagher, R., Graudins, L., Kelly, M., Montomery, J. & Nicholls, G. 2011, Recommendations for terminology, abbreviations and symbols used in the prescribing and administration of medicines. Australian Commission on Safety and Quality in Health Care. http://www.safetyandquality.gov.au/wp -content/uploads/2012/01/32060v2.pdf

Australian Nursing and Midwifery Council 2002, *National competency standards for the enrolled nurse*, viewed 28 June 2015, http:// www.nursingmidwiferyboard.gov.au/Codes -Guidelines-Statements/Codes-Guidelines .aspx#competencystandards

Department of Education, Employment and Workplace Relations 2012, *HLTEN502B Apply effective communication skills in nursing practice*, https://training.gov.au /TrainingComponentFiles/HLT07/HLTEN502B _R1.pdf

Department of Education, Employment and Workplace Relations 2012, *HLTEN504C Implement and evaluate a plan of nursing care*, https://training.gov.au /TrainingComponentFiles/HLT07/HLTEN504C _R1.pdf

Department of Education, Employment and Workplace Relations 2012, *HLTEN509B Apply legal and ethical parameters to nursing practice*, https://training.gov.au /TrainingComponentFiles/HLT07/HLTEN509B _R1.pdf

Department of Education, Employment and Workplace Relations 2012, *HLTOHS300B Contribute to OHS processes*, https://training .gov.au/TrainingComponentFiles/HLT07 /HLTOHS300B_R1.pdf

Department of Education, Employment and Workplace Relations 2012, *HLTEN507C Administer and monitor medications in the work environment*, http://training.gov.au /TrainingComponentFiles/HLT07/HLTEN507C _R1.pdf

Department of Education and Training 2014, *Training.gov.au*, viewed 11 December 2014, http://training.gov.au/Search/Training/

Department of Education and Training 2014, *Training.gov.au. Unit of competency details HLTIN301C - Comply with infection control policies and procedures*, viewed 13 October 2014, http://training.gov.au/Training/Details /HLTEN507C

Jefferies, D., Johnson, M., Nicholls, D. & Lad, S. 2012, A ward-based writing coach program to improve the quality of nursing documentation, *Nurse Education Today*, vol. 32, pp. 647–51.

Society of Hospital Pharmacists of Australia 2014, *Australian injectable drugs handbook* (2014), 6th edn, SHPA, Collingwood Victoria.

Teytelman, Y. 2002. Effective nursing documentation and communication, *Seminars in Oncology Nursing*, vol. 18(12), pp. 121–7.

CHAPTER 4

Alexander, M., Corrigan, A., Gorski, L., Hankins, J. & Perucca, R. (eds) 2010. *Infusion nursing: an evidence-based approach*, Saunders Elservier, St. Louis Missouri.

Broyles, B., Reiss, B., Evans, M., McKenzie, G., Pleunik, S. & Page, R. 2013, *Phamacology in nursing: Australia and New Zealand*, 1st edn, Cengage Learning, South Melbourne Australia.

Gahart, B. & Nazareno, A. 2014, *2015 Intravenous Medications: A Handbook for Nurses and Health Professionals*, MOSBY, Elsevier.

MIMS Australia 2014, MIMS annual.

CHAPTER 5

Australian Commission on Safety and Quality in Health Care 2014, National recommendations for user-applied labelling of injectable medicines, fluids and lines, viewed 26 October 2014, http://www.safetyandquality.gov.au/our-work /medication-safety/safer-naming-labelling-and-packaging-of-medicines/user-applied-labelling/

Brotto, V. & Rafferty, K. 2016. *Clinical Dosage Calculations for Australia and New Zealand*, 2nd edn, Cengage Learning, South Melbourne Australia.

Broyles, B., Reiss, B., Evans, M., McKenzie, G., Pleunik, S. & Page, R. 2013, *Pharmacology in nursing: Australia and New Zealand*, 1st edn, Cengage Learning, South Melbourne Australia.

Department of Education and Training 2014, *Training.gov.au*, viewed 11 December 2014, http://training.gov.au/Search/Training/

National Health and Medical Research Council 2010, *Australian guidelines for the prevention and control of infection in healthcare*, http://www .nhmrc.gov.au/_files_nhmrc/publications /attachments/cd33_complete.pdf

World Health Organization 2009, *WHO guidelines on hand hygiene in health care. First global patient safety challenge clean care is safer care*, World Health Organization Press, Geneva, http://whqlibdoc.who.int /publications/2009/9789241597906_eng.pdf

Wright, K. 2011, *Drug calculations for nurses: context for practice*, Palgrave Macmillan, London.

CHAPTER 6

Australian Commission on Safety and Quality in Health Care 2014, *Paediatric national inpatient medication charts*, viewed 12 December 2014, http://www.safetyandquality.gov.au/our-work /medication-safety/medication-chart/paediatric -medication-charts/

Brotto, V. & Rafferty, K. 2016. *Clinical Dosage Calculations for Australia and New Zealand*, 2nd edn, Cengage Learning, South Melbourne Australia.

Department of Education and Training 2014, *Training.gov.au*, viewed 11 December 2014, http://training.gov.au/Search/Training/

National Health and Medical Research Council (NHMRC) 2014, *Aseptic non-touch technique*, viewed 6 December 2014, http://www.nhmrc .gov.au/book/australian-guidelines-prevention -and-control-infectionhealthcare-2010/b1-7-1 -aseptic-non-touch

Roughead, L., Semple, S. & Rosenfeld, E. 2013, *Literature review: medication safety in Australia*, viewed 8 December 2014, http://www.safetyandquality.gov.au/wp -content/uploads/2014/02/Literature -Review-Medication-Safety-in-Australia -2013.pdf

Society of Hospital Pharmacists of Australia 2014, *Australian injectable drugs handbook* (2014), 6th edn, SHPA, Collingwood Victoria.

APPENDIX B: INTRAVENOUS CARE

Australian Commission on Safety and Quality in Health Care 2012, *National Recommendations for User-applied Labelling of Injectable Medicines, Fluids and Lines*, viewed from http://www.safetyandquality.gov.au /wp-content/uploads/2012/03 /Labelling-Recommendations- 2nd-edition -February-2012.pdf

Centre for Healthcare Related Infection Surveillance and Preventions & Tuberculosis Control (CHRISP&TC) 2013, *Guideline for Peripheral Intravenous Catheters (PIVC)*, viewed from https://www.health.qld.gov .au/qhpolicy/docs/gdl/qh-gdl-321-6-5.pdf

Dougherty, L. & Lister, S. (eds) 2011, *The Royal Marsden Hospital Manual of Clinical Nursing Procedures*, 8th ed., Oxford: Wiley-Blackwell.

Fong, E. 2014, *Peripheral Intravenous Lines: Maintenance*, viewed from Joanna Briggs Institute, http://joannabriggs.org

Joanna Briggs Institute 2013a, *Blood Specimen Collection – Recommended Practice*, viewed from Joanna Briggs Institute, http://joannabriggs.org

Joanna Briggs Institute 2013b, *Intravenous Therapy: Infusion Pumps Recommended Practices*, viewed from Joanna Briggs Institute, http://joannabriggs.org

Perry, A. G. & Potter, P. A. 2006, *Clinical Nursing Skills and Techniques*, 6th ed., St Louis, Missouri: Mosby.

Sayakkara, S. 2014, *Phlebitis: Risk Assessment*, viewed from Joanna Briggs Institute, http://joannabriggs.org

Slade, S. 2013, *Evidence Summary: Blood Specimen Collection: Haemolysis Prevention*, viewed from Joanna Briggs Institute, http://joannabriggs.org

INDEX